THE DISCOVERY OF JJ'S WAY

YOUR BASIC GUIDE TO 20 POUNDS IN 12 WEEKS

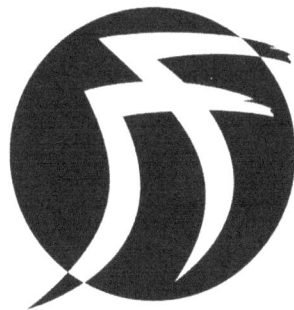

JJFM Productions

Cover art and design by Mquad Design, LLC.

JJFitness and its logo, two intersecting letters "J" encircled, are trademarks of JJFitnessMedia Productions.

Visit our website at www.jjfitness.net

ISBN 978-0-6151-9068-6

THE DISCOVERY OF JJ'S WAY

Your Basic Guide to 20 pounds in 12 weeks

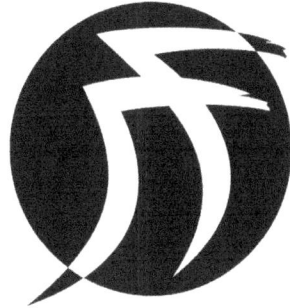

Introduction

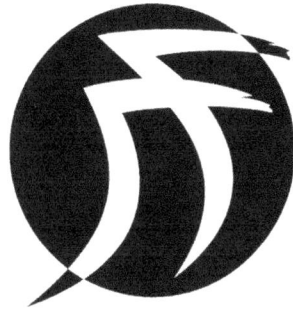

I remember it like it was 10 minutes ago.

I'm at my gym, a small, private training facility that lets a few dedicated people work out on their own.

I'm sitting on an upright bench, resting between sets of a hard workout.

The owner of the gym is having a friendly disagreement with a friend on the phone.

"Hey JJ!" he calls from his office.

I look over and nod.

"Me and my man got a bet about body weight and squatting."

"What's that?" I say, suddenly interested.

"He's trying to tell me that as a guy gets closer to 300 pounds, it gets harder and harder to squat over 400. He says your body weight prevents it!"

"What's that got to do with me?"

"You're pretty close to 300 aren't you?"

I don't answer. What in the heck is this guy talking about? Stunned, like I've just been blindsided with a big left hook in the temple, I turn back to look at the mirrors.

I have to admit, I still kind of like what I am seeing. I have big broad shoulders and sizeable biceps...(little did I know till later that it was some muscle covered by a lot of "extra").

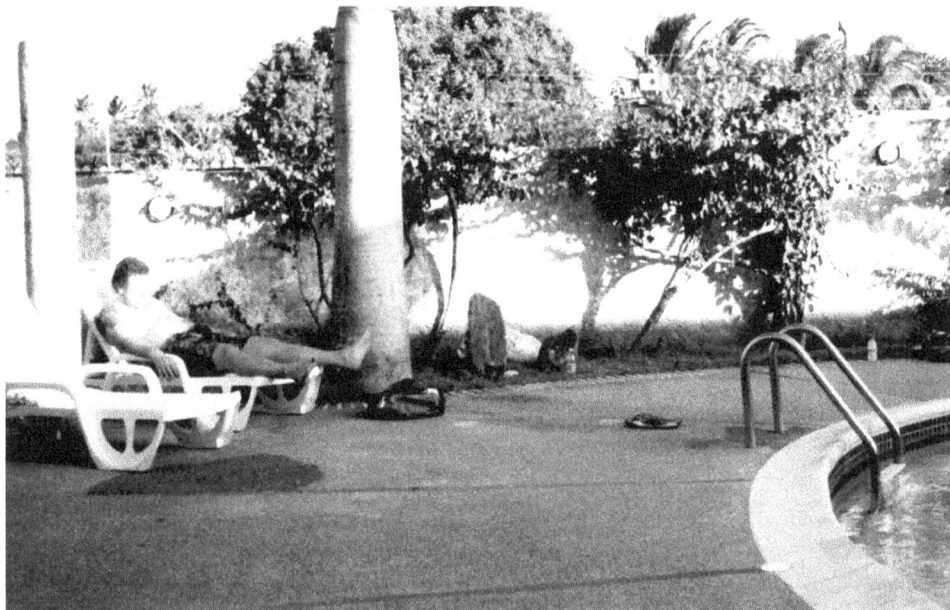

I am in my prime! (or so I thought....)

I've written and published a novel, am finishing my academic graduate work and teaching at an elite institution, I travel all over the world for conferences and seminars. I work out 3-5 times a week, have great friends and enjoy my easygoing lifestyle.

'This guy must be trying to mess with my head,' I say to myself, smiling. 'Imagine that! A gym rat who wears a grey sweat suit and work boots every day trying to get in the head of one of the best up and coming philosophers in the game! HA!'

In reality, I don't know what to do. My enthusiasm for finishing my workout has completely flown out the window.

'At any rate,' I think, 'I'm not going to let my ego get in the way here. He works with body builders and power lifters for a living, so he must be seeing something. And this dude is a real stoic, so I don't think he's just goofing around.'

I remove my shoes, sweatshirt, and sweatpants, and go to the scale in the back of the gym. I take a deep breath, and step on.

Unbelievably, shockingly, the scale reads **275 pounds**.

On this very day, I experienced <u>my</u> "LIGHTBULB" moment. From that instant, when I saw that number - the number that represented how much excess weight I was carrying - my life changed. It stays with me always.

I immediately scheduled an appointment with my doctor. When my tests came back, **my fasting blood sugar was 146**. My fasting level should have been 110 or less. **I was pre-diabetic!**

I knew very well what could happen with diabetes - all the injections, the loss of my foot or leg - and I was right on the road to that reality.

When I asked my doctor what I could do, the answer I got was so general and vague, "eat a healthy diet and exercise" that I left his office probably in the most disappointed state I've ever been in.

I asked myself, HOW DID I GET LIKE THIS? I worked out and I didn't eat a crazy amount. True, I did enjoy my share of pizzas, cheese steaks, pasta, but I rarely ate sweets. I had a few beers now and again but nothing too out of control. And here I was on the edge of a serious health problem.

Not too mention the way I ACTUALLY looked, which was NOT HOT.

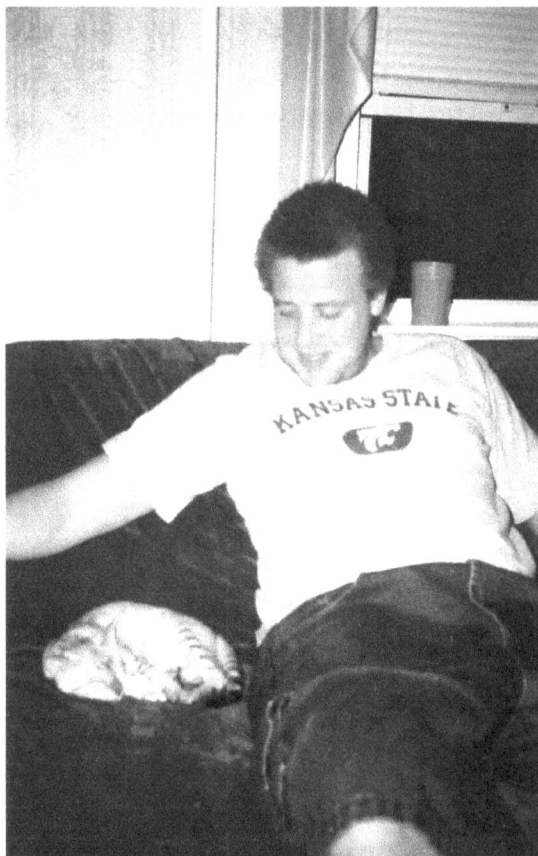

I knew I needed help right away. As a 'thank you' for turning on the light bulb in my life, my first positive act was to hire that same gym owner for a short time to help me, and I went into training. This invaluable time with a master trainer gave me a blueprint to follow, during which time I began a tireless research effort at my university library and the local bookstores.

Like a person possessed, I read about all the systems of training and types of dieting that I could find. We all know how much there is of that! So much that when I finished up my dissertation I went to work full time on the most worthy project of all - myself.

Introduction

I began incorporating the best parts of what I learned into my training and my lifestyle. If something worked and was healthy, I kept it, if it didn't seem be effective, or if it was effective but wasn't part of a healthy lifestyle (ephedrine, for example), it did not have a place in my life. I kept trying and never let anything deter me from my goal weight - 200 pounds. I knew that weight comes off the same way it goes on...one pound at a time.

This is how JJ's Way was Discovered.

One tough year later, I had lost 1/4 of my body weight.

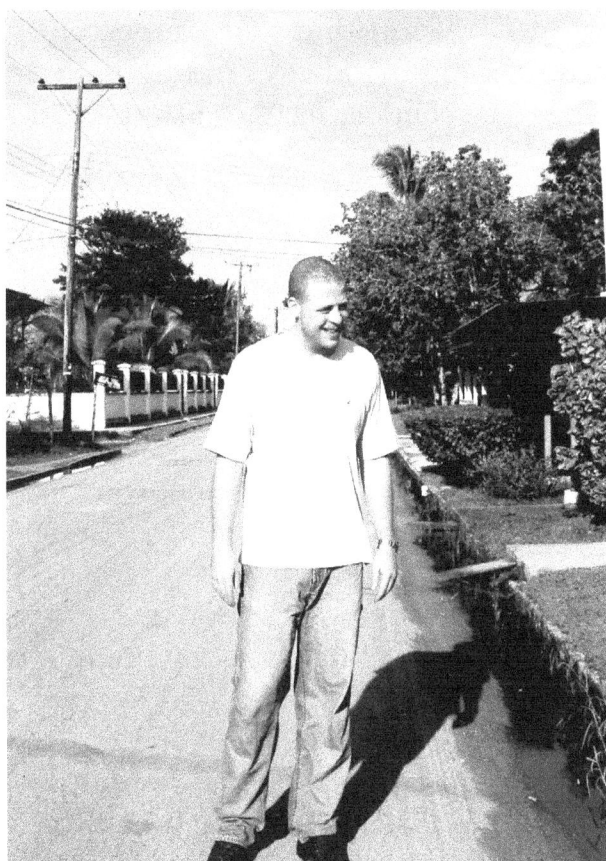

Looking back, my de-conditioned, obese state was not all that atypical. America is full of people who are much more overweight than they realize. Some even believe they're fit. Others may recognize they're out of shape. Most haven't got a clue what to do about it.

When it came to food, like many it was for me always the procrastination of "I'll start tomorrow."

When I looked in the mirror, I rationalized "I don't look so bad. Not great, but not too bad. I can still get around well and I work long days."

Deep down I knew I was fooling myself. I had to turn things around.

I had several advantages in my favor: first, because I was a graduate student at the time I could lead a very scheduled, almost secluded life that allowed me to NEVER miss on my diet and avoid all temptations to stray.

Secondly, I had been a college athlete. That gave me a certain advantage in resistance training, but more importantly I knew about the benefits of discipline and not always indulging in immediate gratification of things like comfort food and that extra hour of television.

That being said, everyone has their own set of advantages. It is very important to identify them and "take advantage of your advantages." If you are a stay at home mom, use the fact that you run your own schedule. If you work in an office, find a gym nearby that you like and check it out during a break. Whatever your situation is, whether you have been fit in the past and are looking for a way to get it back, or you have never set foot on a gym floor in your life, work it and make it work!

It was near the end of my first year of JJ's Way training that I decided to leave the academic profession and take my life in a different, more positive direction.

As I achieved my goal weight, I was blessed to find my life passion for fitness and my complete dedication to being a health care professional. Since then I have helped a lot of people get more fit, more healthy, more well, and more happy.

As I continued with my research, I realized that we are in the middle of a <u>real, full blown epidemic</u> in this country,

We need to work together to eradicate the American obesity epidemic before there is a widespread health crisis.

And it starts with YOU.

You know how JJ's Way was discovered. Now I want to help you discover it as well, but more importantly, discover yourself!

I believe that JJ's Way can help you can achieve a profound transformation!

Even though the particulars of my situation are no doubt different than yours, I am no different than you. I'm not one of those fitness freaks that have always been in shape and look perfect and can't identify with the struggle you are going through.

If I did it, you can too.

THIS IS WHAT THE GAME IS ABOUT....
You hang in there,
Overcome disappointments,
Overcome injuries,
You keep believing,
You don't get down.
When it looks bleak,
You hang in there and KEEP FIGHTING

The thing that changes your life forever
could be right on the next page...

Chapter 1: Red or Green Pill?

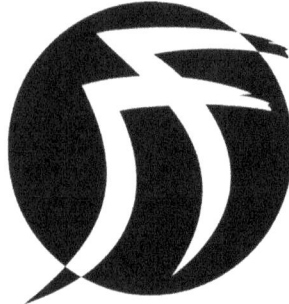

If you have more than 20 pounds of weight to lose, you have an important decision to make.

It may be a vanity decision
It may be a quality of life decision
It may be a life and death decision

WHAT ARE YOUR CHOICES?

In each hand you have a pill. In one hand, red, in the other, green.

If you take the <u>red pill, nothing happens</u>, you go on living in the same compromised state of health and fitness as you are now. The same look, weight, the same strength, the same fluctuating energy level. You have back pain and probably plenty of other places that hurt.

You either have diabetes, high blood pressure, and heart disease or are in danger of them.

The red pill is the Stay-the-Same Pill, keeping you in what we call *Stasis*.

BUT, when you take the <u>green pill, you start seeing consistent, dramatic change</u>!

Right Away, you are stronger, more in balance, you're moving better with more confidence.

Your back pain decreases and probably disappears altogether!

Within two weeks, your friends say they notice you look better.

Within three weeks, your pants don't fit as tight. You don't have to hold your breath to get them on or zip them!

In two short months, your energy is greatly improved and you even look forward to sweating 3 or 4 times a week.

In 12 weeks, please believe it, you have lost 20 pounds or more. The green pill is the *Change Pill*.

ASK YOURSELF RIGHT NOW: Which one would you take?

RED PILL (stasis) GREEN PILL (change)

RED is STOP...GREEN is GO!

JJ's Way is your Green Pill

A JJ's Way Experience

When I first considered what need to be different in my life to become healthier, I wondered if I would be disciplined enough to make the changes that mattered and keep making them. After all, there is something comfortable about the familiar, like eating ice cream when stressed, and in that respect, the red pill seemed to have its purpose.

In spite of desire to stay within my "comfort" zone, there was an ongoing battle in my mind between the two pills.

When I took a step back and looked objectively at my life, taking the red pill really made my life more unmanageable and stressful, especially when I stepped on the scale wondering if my weight stayed the same or went up depending on my habits, or when I had to lay on the bed to get on my "stretch" pants!

I found that I was avoiding a lot more than just losing weight by continuing my unhealthy ways.

It was a success for me to even start JJ's Way, and once I did, I learned I needed the structure of a meal and exercise plan in order to make better decisions for myself. I found that discipline is something that develops over time, and not all at once. JJ's program helped me to connect with strengths that I didn't know I had!

Food has lost most of its emotional meaning for me and I now am more motivated to eat because my body needs energy because of my high activity level rather than for other reasons.

I've lost 60 pounds and several clothing sizes, and I gained a lot more than what I lost in terms of self respect, confidence, and good health. I'm not "perfect" in terms of my eating and following through on my workouts, but I am "good enough" to have achieved those results!

Stephanie S., JJFitness Charter Member

Precautions Before Beginning an Exercise Program

Consult a physician before starting any resistance exercise and before beginning JJ's Way Lifestyle

See a physical or occupational therapist beforehand if you have musculoskeletal pain

Expect soreness at the beginning of any new exercise program

Contact your doctor is you have severe soreness (deep ache and unusual stiffness) for more than 3 days after a workout

Listen to your body. Pain is a signal that something is wrong. Follow up immediately with a medical professional

Chapter 2: The Good Stuff

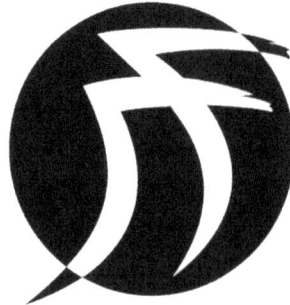

This fitness book is different from any other fitness book: it will give to you the thing that can't be bought or paid for.

What is that? Self Discovery!

YOU and YOU ALONE are in charge of what happens in this story.

There are challenges, choices, adventures and consequences. YOU must use all of your wits and your intelligence. An ill informed decision, like consistent overeating or smoking cigarettes, could end in severe consequences – even death. But, don't despair. At any time, YOU can go back and make another choice, alter the path of your story, and change its result. You write the ending to this story.

YOU may lose that first 20 pounds for the last time, never to return.

YOU will enter the fun and challenging world of fitness.

Whatever happens, you will learn a lot about yourself, what you're capable of accomplishing, and no matter what, you'll be taking that first important step towards health and fitness.

Good luck!

It's Your Adventure.

You are here because there is a discovery to be made, the most important discovery:

The Self-Discovery of your health and fitness!

But the Discovery cannot be given to you. You will have to make some choices.

But First, here are a few questions we can answer right away:

How many times a week will I be exercising? 3-4

What is the eating plan like? Simple, Healthy and Easy to follow

How much cardio do I have to do? Not too much, not too hard. Less Is More!

Will I be lifting weights? Yes! Resistance Training is the key to every sustainable weight loss effort.

How difficult is this? Challenging, but you <u>can</u> do it!

Your Body is a Reflection of YOU!

Your success in weight loss depends more on your lifestyle and your attitude
than what you do working out.

Please take a few minutes to answer these three questions:

1. How do I describe myself?

2. How do I describe my ideal self?

3. What is ONE thing I can start doing today to get closer to my ideal self?

Chapter 3: Is It In You?

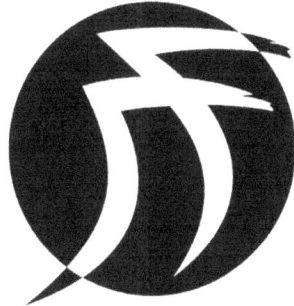

JJ's Way is a real and continuing challenge.

This is because your body is constantly seeking the red pill - a state of stasis.

But stasis is actually impossible.

You are always moving either closer or farther away from your healthiest being. Which direction you choose is up to you.

Let's get clear: the green pill is NOT the "easy" pill, but it does get easier as time passes. As you follow the plan, you begin to intuitively adapt to a healthier lifestyle. You will Discover that being healthy is actually more simple and manageable than you think.

"IT'S NOT A CHANCE UNLESS YOU TAKE IT!"

The Discovery Phase of JJ's Way is not complicated or unrealistic:

The Goal is to live a healthy lifestyle for 12 weeks and lose your first 20 pounds or more.

It won't be easy, and putting yourself out there to try something that is not a sure thing is definitely a risk.
But remember this – ALL EXPLORERS TAKE RISKS.

BUT are you _ready_ for _change_?

Everybody wants to change something about themselves. There are very few people who WOULDN'T want to take off 20 pounds or more…such is the American lifestyle. Nearly all of us are at least somewhat overweight. But how many are ready to do what's really necessary to make that change?

Are you ready?

We can determine that by using a model called the Stages of Change. How ready you are to manage your weight depends on what Stage of Change you are in.

The Stages of Change are:
> **Pre-contemplation**
> **Contemplation**
> **Preparation**
> **Action**
> **Maintenance**
> **Termination**

If you don't believe you have a weight problem or do not want to lose weight despite being overweight, then you are in **Precontemplation**.

If you are considering losing weight or starting an exercise program, then you are in **Contemplation**.

If you have picked a start date to begin losing weight or exercising then you are in **Preparation**.

When you have begun your plan you are in **Action**.

When you have reached your goals, you then work to prevent relapse of unhealthy behaviors and maintain your current weight and fitness level in the **Maintenance** stage.

It is very important to remember that these stages are not linear! It is very common to go back and forth between the first 3, like a spiral, before moving through. Even in the Action or Maintenance phase, it is possible to return to the initial stages.

What are the Stages of Change for Health & Fitness?

Stage	Characteristics
Pre-contemplation	• Not admitting the problem • Not considering change
Contemplation	• Aware of the problem • Thinking about change • Unsure if change is a good idea. • Uncertain about how to go about change
Preparation	• Gathering information about how to make change • Ready to learn • Developing coping skills to change • Considering options: easy way / hard way • Red or Green Pill?
Action	• The simple act of doing! • Starting to take the Green Pill • Translating information into action • Practice at least 6 months • Just like when you were learning to drive a car, you had to pay attention and practice so you didn't get into an accident
Maintenance	• Change is more natural / automatic • Practice AND Reinforcement • You passed your driver's test and are a good driver • You have met most of your goals • Routine • The search for mastery begins

These stages are not linear....but instead like a horizontal spiral.

Change is not just behavioral

Change is also emotional and cognitive

Change is a PROCESS

**Stages of Change:
Self-Assessment Worksheet**

Circle the statements which apply to you:

PRE-CONTEMPLATION

◊ I don't want to be in training
◊ The way I eat is healthy and I'm doing fine
◊ I enjoy my current lifestyle and will continue

CONTEMPLATION

◊ I need to change my lifestyle to become more fit and healthy
◊ Changing my eating habits will be difficult. I'll miss my favorites like cake and pizza. Creating time to cook will be a challenge
◊ Comfort foods are big in my life
◊ My life will change once I'm in training and eating well
◊ I am working to accept those changes

PREPARATION

◊ I know specifically what I have to do to change while training and eating well
◊ My significant other and friends know I'm in training and eating well

ACTION

◊ I am eating well
◊ I am training hard
◊ I am aware that fitness takes time and is a process

MAINTENANCE

◊ I hit all my workouts and ate well every day this month
◊ Working out and eating well was a "given" this past week
◊ I am a highly competent trainee
◊ I am training on my own and check in with a fitness consultant occasionally to modify workouts and improve performance

So now we know what Stage of Change you are in. Since you are reading this book, most likely it is Contemplation or Preparation. Congrats…you've taken the very challenging first step in the discovery of JJ's Way!

So how do we get started?

Let's begin by devoting some time to yourself. The most valuable resource you have is time.

For the next 12 weeks, every day you will devote enough time to yourself to live by JJ's Way.

If you make a time commitment to a lifestyle of regular training, you will reap untold benefits.

Is It In You?

YES!

Great, we've made the most important determination: What's next?

Let's figure out what we need to get started – a Discovery kit that will have all the tools and materials we need to begin this adventure.

Chapter 4: The Bare Necessities

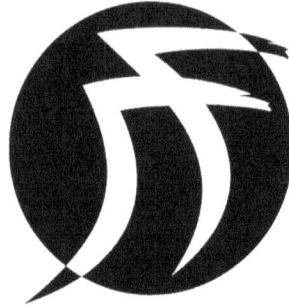

Your Discovery Toolkit

To get started on your journey of Discovery, you will need the following:

<u>Access to basic cardio equipment</u>

No, taking a walk around your neighborhood won't get it done! Cardio equipment will help ensure both Consistency and Proper Intensity.

Examples of acceptable cardio equipment include:
- ➢ Treadmill
- ➢ Exercise Bike
- ➢ Arc Trainer

Where the cardio equipment is - in your home, a local gym, school, work, a friends house, or the local YMCA - does not matter as long as you have consistent access to it.

<u>Heart Rate Monitor (HRM)</u>
A heart rate monitor is a watch with a strap that goes around your chest. For now forget all the calorie counting options and workout programmability. These cost extra money and take up too much time. All you really need is the ability to monitor your heart rate. Nike sells one for under 70 dollars and Polar is slightly more.

Your Discovery Toolkit *(continued)*

Is the HRM absolutely necessary?
You can begin if you have access to a treadmill with heart rate handles, but eventually you will need a Heart Rate Monitor, which will also serve as your timer during your workouts. I guarantee it is the best money you will spend.

Swiss Ball
These come in three sizes. 55cm (small) 65(med/large) 75cm (extra large). Most people will get a 55 or 65cm.

Resistance Bands
I prefer the bands with plastic handles. Roughly 10-12 bucks a piece. You'll need four: yellow, green, red and blue.

Dumbbell weights up to 20 pounds
You will need pairs of 2.5 lb, 7.5 lb, 10 lb, 12 lb, 15 lb, 17 lb and 20 lb dumbbells.

If you are at a gym that has all of these, that will work out best, you would only have to invest in the HRM, ball and elastic bands. If not, go to a local sporting goods store, or gym supply for the bands. Target and Sears now have fantastic fitness sections.

Shoes
Cross-trainers or basketball shoes are best for lateral stability. Gym shoes regularly need to be replaced at least twice a year.

Food scale and Measuring cups
You can find both these items at your local grocery store. You will use these primarily for weighing/measuring out protein and carb portions. As you gain experience you will become better at eyeballing your appropriate portions, but the scale is still useful especially when trying new foods.

Chapter 5: Discovery Journal

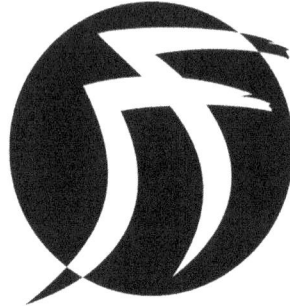

Every good explorer needs a journal. Your journal will be a record of your success, and a guidebook for the future of your health and fitness.

We usually use the Composition notebooks that are roughly 5 x 9. They can be found at any office supply for store for a couple of dollars. If you already keep a journal it would be best to keep your fitness journal in a separate book – it will get beat up, sweated and spilled on, and dirty. Exploring is a rough and tumble adventure!

On the inside cover of your new Discovery Journal write down your name and phone number. You'd be surprised how many workout books get left on treadmills and weight benches.

On the first page, write this:

> ### Get Today Right!

You should feel free to jot down any sayings, tips, instructions and inspirations that will remind and motivate you. This is your journal.

The main purpose of the Discovery journal is to keep track of your workouts and nutrition. I want you to record the date, duration and location of every workout session.

A typical entry might look like this:

> *Week 1 Day 3*
> *Jan 31, 2008*
> *Workout location: Home*
>
> *Workout:*
>
> *DB Chest Press: 7.5 pounds*
> *Band Flye: yellow/green bands*
> *Band Squat: free squat, yellow band*
> *Band Curls: yellow/green bands*
> *Pushups: 6*
>
> *Comments:*
> *Side bends are difficult. Felt stiff and couldn't hold the position.*
> *Quad extensions felt easy... hope I'm doing them right.*

If you have a great workout, a bad workout, reach a goal, or need to record your food intakes, the Discovery Journal is the place to write it down.

Take a few minutes to answer the following question in your Journal:

> *What is motivating me to lose weight and be healthier?*

Your answers might include:
Your looks, the added activities you'll be able to do, added confidence, pride, attention and praise from others, more energy, strength.

The reasons for wanting to become healthy and fit should be encouraging and keep you encouraged.

Let's get the tough stuff out of the way. Measure the following body parts with a tape measure and write them in your Discovery Journal:

Shoulders:

Chest:

Waist:

Hips:

Mid Thigh (right):

Upper Arm (right):

Wrist (right):

In the morning before you've eaten, step on the scale and write down your weight in your Discovery Journal.

Finally, I recommend that you take two pictures of yourself, one from the front and one from the side. Print out the pictures. Next, try to find an older photo of yourself when you were less overweight. Tape all the pictures in your Journal. If you can print an extra photo, I highly recommend that you put one on your refrigerator as well.

I realize that the tasks on this page may feel cumbersome or difficult for you to do. Be strong and get them all done at once - the numbers are just a baseline, a starting point from which you will progress towards your ***true self***.

Chapter 6: What's Your Magic Number?

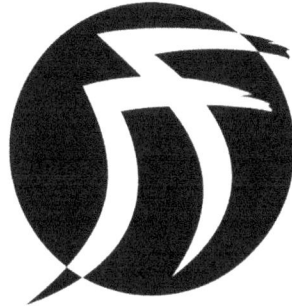

The Treadmill Test

Yes, this is a test. But everybody passes!

This test collects a TREASURE OF INFORMATION about your HEART and LUNGS that is the cornerstone of losing that first 20 pounds.

All your cardiovascular work will be done in heart rate "Zones". There are 5 Zones ranging from "1" (easy) to "5" (very intense).

Read over this entire test before you start to prepare yourself and your Discovery Journal

Make sure your HRM is on and working properly.

There are 2 rules for the treadmill

1. Remember that you are on a treadmill, so don't fall off

2. No Holding On. You may keep one hand on a side rail for balance if needed.

Holding on is a treadmill violation. It allows you to rest part of your weight on the handrails. When you're on the treadmill, it's important for your muscles to support your entire bodyweight. Consider holding on a form of "cheating".

DON'T VIOLATE THE TREADMILL!

Copy the chart below into your Discovery Journal.

	TIME	SPEED	INCLINE
Warm-up	5 min	2.0 – 2.5	2.0
Interval 1	2 min	2.5 – 3.0	4.0
Interval 2	2 min	2.5 – 3.0	6.0
Interval 3	2 min	2.5 – 3.5	8.0
Cool-down	5 min	2.0	2.0

Start the treadmill and keep it on manual setting.

Begin by setting your incline to 2.0 and speed to 2.0 for 5 minutes. (For all levels of fitness, this is how each workout should be started)

This is Zone 1, the warm-up zone. During this time, your core temperature rises and your nervous system prepares to gear up. You should not notice any big difference in breathing at this time.

If you do notice that there is significant change in your breathing during warm-up, that is ok. Write it in your Discovery Journal! Otherwise in 12 weeks, you won't believe yourself when you look back.

After 5 minutes:

Move the speed up so that you're moving slightly (not too much) faster. I want you to be at a medium paced walk. Try 2.5 and see how that feels, if it feels 'too cold' go for the 'just right of 2.7 or 2.9'

Move the incline up to 4.0

Walk for two minutes.

What is your heart rate? Write it down.

Remember: NO HOLDING ON!

Holding on is a *treadmill violation*.

If you are De-conditioned, you will notice significant changes in your breathing here. Press on!

You are most likely now in Zone 2. Believe it or not, **this is your most efficient fat burning Zone.**

After 2 minutes, keep the same speed and move the incline up to 6.0

Ouch? You may feel a slight burning in your calves....this is because you are De-conditioned. Press on a little bit longer.

The data you are collecting is a valuable treasure!

What is your Heart Rate? Write it down. You are most likely now in Zone 3.

If you are 'out of breath' or feel burning in your thighs or booty, write down your HR and move down to incline 2.0 and speed 2.0

OK, if you are breathing hard but not totally out of breath, lets go up to incline 8 for one final push.

We are seeking your Threshold.

The Threshold is the point at which you basically stop burning fat.

You are at your threshold if:
You 'have to' breathe through your mouth
A complete sentence is only possible with two breaths
You feel burning in your thighs and/or booty.

When you reach this point, note your HR number, and move down to incline 2.0 and speed 2.0.

Always cool down for 5 minutes at incline 2.0 and speed 2.0

CONGRATS, you are done, and it thankfully it won't be this hard again for 3 or 4 weeks at least!

AND it was worth it! You have successfully discovered your most important TREASURE. Your Magic number for your Anaerobic Threshold (AT).

Your Threshold number is like your cardio fingerprint.

Record Your Threshold in the <u>My AT</u> box of the "Weeks 1-4" column on the next page. You should also write your AT in your Discovery Journal.

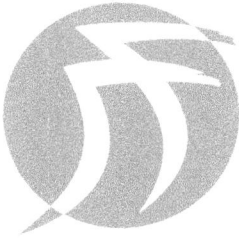

JJFitness My Zones

	Weeks 1 - 4	Weeks 5 - 8	Weeks 9 - 12
	Deconditioned	*Transitional*	*Conditioned*
Date of Test			
My AT			
My Zone 1			
My Zone 2			
My Zone 3			
My Zone 4			
My Zone 5			

But you can't work out at your AT every time you do cardio! In fact, you won't be getting anywhere near your AT again for quite a while.

So let's look at which heart rates you'll be working out. Find your AT number in the left column on the next page. The horizontal column to the right of your number tells you the heart rate range of your Zones. Come back to your JJFitness My Zones chart on this page and write each of your zones in the Weeks 1-4 column. Test again on Week 5, and again on Week 9. Using your Zones will be critical when you begin the JJFitness Cardio routines on pg. 79 of this book.

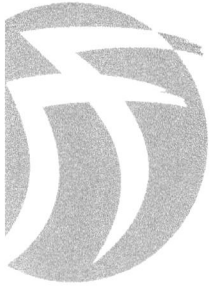

JJFitness Zone Finder

Anerobic Threshold	Zone 1 Warm up/Cool down *Easy*	Zone 2 Fat Loss *Medium*	Zone 3 Aerobic Endurance *Hard*	Zone 4 Anaerobic Endurance *Very Hard*	Zone 5 Speed/Power *Extremely Har*
120	72 - 84	84 - 108	108 - **120**	120 - 132	132 - ma
125	75 - 88	88 - 113	113 - 125	125 - 138	138 - ma
130	78 - 91	91 - 117	117 - 130	130 - 143	143 - ma
135	81 - 95	95 - 122	122 - 135	135 - 149	149 - ma
140	84 - 98	98 - 126	126 - 140	140 - 154	154 - ma
145	87 - 102	102 - 131	131 - 145	145 - 160	160 - ma
150	90 - 105	105 - 136	135 - 150	150 - 165	165 - ma
155	93 - 109	109 - 140	140 - 155	155 - 171	171 - ma
160	96 - 112	112 - 144	144 - 160	160 - 176	176 - ma
165	99 - 116	116 - 149	149 - 165	165 - 182	182 - ma
170	102 - 119	119 - 153	153 - 170	170 - 187	187 - ma
175	105 - 123	123 - 158	158 - 175	175 - 193	193 - ma
180	108 - 126	126 - 162	162 - 180	180 - 198	198 - ma
185	111 - 130	130 - 167	167 - 185	185 - 204	204 - ma
190	114 - 133	133 - 171	171 - 190	190 - 209	209 - ma
195	117 - 136	137 - 176	176 - 195	195 - 214	214 - ma
200	120 - 139	140 - 180	180 - 200	200 - 219	219 - ma

Zone 2 Workout: Contrary to popular belief, most good fat burning is done in a moderate heart rate zone. You'll be spending most of your time during these first 12 weeks (and beyond) in a mid to high Zone 2. Because it builds an aerobic base, so do most elite endurance athletes!

Some physical signs you are in Zone 2:

◊ You feel like you could go faster/harder
◊ You can talk in complete sentences without breaking to breathe
◊ You can breathe through your nose
◊ More sweat than usual…a slow burn feeling.

After working out in Zone 2, your body will still feel fresh, little to no stress, you will have energy and not feel tired/burned out, and you will be burning fat for hours to come. It's truly the best of both worlds!

Interval Workout: An interval workout conditions your body by stepping up into Zone 3 for short periods of time, then using Zone 2 to recover. An Interval workout is a great workout to get fit in a short time, and because it is more intense will burn a lot of fat. That does NOT mean that you should do it more often. More is not better.

Some Physical signs you are in Zone 3:

◊ You feel like you are at a strong/difficult workout pace
◊ You need to take a break to breathe while talking

There is a lot of information in this next chapter.
It is probably the most important part of this book.
Read as much as you can and then move to page 48 for the good stuff.

You can come back later for more info and motivation

Chapter 7: Are You Heavy, Tired, and Depressed?

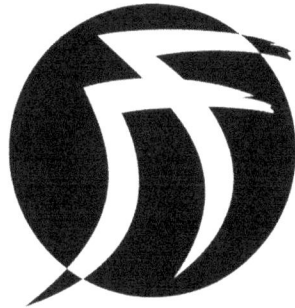

Why haven't other diets worked before?

Can YOU really become fit, healthy, well?

> **HERE'S THE "LIGHTBULB" MOMENT YOU'VE BEEN WAITING FOR:**
>
> *You didn't gain weight simply because you are lazy or lack self-control!*

Most diets focus on restricting food intake – carefully, obsessively watching calories! In fact, because of its effect on metabolism most calorie restriction contributes to eventual weight gain. Popular shows like The Biggest Loser give the idea that calorie counting is the way to lose a lot of weight fast. But The Biggest Loser isn't "real", it's good entertainment…everything the TV producers do behind the scenes is for that "wow" moment when the contestants step on the scale. They keep the Losers in a carefully controlled environment, and work them near to death with excessively intense workouts that make the trainees highly susceptible to injury. They do lose weight, but it far from healthy. Check in on a Biggest Loser contestant 5 years after they've been on the show and see what their real results are…

You need a plan you can live for the rest of your life.

JJ's Way knows that obesity is not from overeating alone – taking in too many calories – but mostly from the body's use of *Sugars and Starches* for making fat.

Simply put, it's more chemical than quantity:

 What you eat makes much more of a difference than _how much_ you eat

Almost everyone "mis-metabolizes" Sugars and Starches. They actually cause a disturbance in how your body runs.

And when there's a disturbance in your metabolism, there are 3 Results, none of them good for you!

    Result 1. your body *forms fat faster* than normal
    Result 2. your body *stores fat faster* than normal
    Result 3. your body *disposes of stored fat slower* than normal

Don't rely on the counting calories!

You don't lose weight measuring food like you measure energy:

→calories in (eating)← vs. ←calories out (burning)→

because

NOT all calories are the same

So:

Calorie counting is NOT
the best way
to get control
of your weight

The MOST IMPORTANT THING is not how many calories you take in, but what *your* body, not anyone else's body, does with those calories.

> **Food** entering your body is a lot like the words spoken in someone's ear at the beginning of the Telephone Game. Because of enzymes, hormones, energy cycles and many lifestyle factors, it's a real challenge to predict the fate of a particular piece of food on your weight.

The Bottom Line:
The fat from that bacon you ate at breakfast does not end up directly on your hips or stomach. It just doesn't work that way.

But almost ALL of the calories from the Sugars and Starches you eat ends up stored as fat.

Hey, wait a minute!

What about that skinny guy you know who eats pizza every night? Or the model who swears by a diet of ice cream and French bread?

Well: everyone is REALLY DIFFERENT in their ability to "burn" calories as opposed to "save them, whether their body says "stay" to some foods and "go" to others. Skinny Pizza guy and Model Ice Cream girl are rare exceptions to a rule. It's the same reason everyone is not 6'10" and can jump 4 feet high.

I wish I could eat Spaghetti Bolognese and drink beer every night and stay at my fighting weight.
> But I can't!!!

That being said, there is A LOT you can do to turn the tide in your favor.

Here is the truth:

SUGARS and STARCHES are far more responsible for obesity than fat is.

The BIG FAT Lie

The big fat lie says that calorie counting and a no-fat diet are the best way to lose weight.

The no-fat and calorie counting industry emerged for one reason:

To sell you no-fat, processed foods!

The big fat lie has led to people actually gaining weight and living less healthy lives.

Your body cannot live without taking in protein and fat, but has no real need for Sugars and Starches. You don't have to live without them, but it is important to remember that you don't HAVE to have them to live.

Sugars and Starches form the least valuable part of your diet.

They contribute nothing that you can't get better from fat and protein foods like meat, fish, eggs and cheese, plus lots of green vegetables, a little fruit, and unrefined whole grains.

Protein, lots of veggies, a little fruit, a dash of unrefined carbohydrates. This is essentially **JJ's Way** to Health and Wellness

The Nitty Gritty

What happens in your body when you eat food?

Why do some people store everything as fat and others don't?

What determines whether what you eat goes on your hips or is burned up as energy?

The ANSWER to all these questions is the same: **HORMONES**

Hormones control everything that happens in your body: they are the air traffic controllers of you!

And YOU control the air traffic controllers with lifestyle decisions.

Food – along with exercise, stress and rest – is what stimulates some hormones and not others.

Hormones direct your body to store or burn fat.

If the food you eat stimulates the wrong hormones and creates an unbalanced state it is *difficult if not impossible to lose weight* or keep it off.

That is why:

Food is the most powerful drug you will ever encounter

It causes dramatic changes in your hormones that are a hundred times more powerful and more consistent than anything from the drugstore or street corner. But unlike drugs, food is necessary for life, so you have constant contact with it and have to make the right decisions about what to take in and not to take in to stay healthy.

It is all-important to balance your hormones if you want to lose weight. Let's meet these actors.

INTRODUCING: Your Hormones!

The star of the show: **INSULIN**

Insulin is an anabolic hormone. Anabolic hormones are builders, they put compounds like amino acids (protein) and glucose (sugars) inside storage units (cells).

Insulin is released when blood sugar is high, causing liver and muscle cells to take in and store sugar, and causing fat cells to take in blood lipids and turn them into fat.

You cannot survive without insulin, but you can live A LOT better without too much insulin.

Insulin is directly responsible for many chronic illnesses.
obesity, diabetes, heart disease,
hypertension,
polycystic ovary syndrome,
inflammatory diseases,
certain cancers.

There are two basic ways to raise insulin levels.
1. Eat too much Sugar and Starch.
2. Eat too much food.

<u>Most Americans do both!</u>

An overload of insulin is the reason for almost all fat storage and retention.

"IT'S MORE CHEMICAL THAN QUANTITY!"

Normalizing your blood sugar and insulin
response is the main goal of limiting your Sugar and Starch intake, and is THE most important key to weight loss.

The co-star: GLUCAGON

Glucagon is a catabolic hormone. It is a deconstructor, opening up cells and releasing contents as your body needs it.

Glucagon is released when the sugar level in the blood is low, causing your liver to convert stored sugar and release it into the bloodstream.

Both Insulin and Glucagon are released by the pancreas in response to food intakes or absence.

Insulin is a saver, Glucagon is a spender.

Together their job is to maintain a safe range of blood sugar to keep the metabolism running smoothly.

Just like in Star Wars, the dark side (insulin) and the force (glucagon) do a constant dance in your body.

The Air Control Tower: **YOUR PANCREAS**

Insulin is the powerhouse of the pancreatic hormones. It requires FIVE hormones – glucagon, cortisol, adrenaline, nor-adrenaline, and human growth hormone (HGH) – to counterbalance its effects.

The Pancreas is like the tower at an airport. When a plane is coming in to land, the folks inside the tower decide which air traffic controller to deploy onto the runway to ensure a proper landing. When food enters the body, the Pancreas determines which and how much hormone to send into the bloodstream.

Fat doesn't even trigger a "lights on" signal from the pancreas. It has no impact on insulin release.

Protein gets a friendly "all clear for landing" from the pancreas, it secretes a small amount of insulin into the bloodstream

When **Sugars and Starches** pass through, the pancreas brings out the **big guns** onto the airstrip and goes to town, secreting large amounts of insulin into your blood stream.

To fix an immediate problem (sugar in the blood) your body is forced to bring in artillery (insulin), even though in the long run the effects may be devastating, messing up the runways, clogging the terminal, jamming the parking lot.

The liver then converts sugar into stored fat.

Excess levels of insulin is like having a loose cannon firing on the runway of your airport!

The CYCLE OF OBESITY

Sugar and Starch are much more damaging to the body than Fat.

Insulin is the winner of the triple crown:

I. Insulin is the fat storage hormone. It moves fat into cells and keeps it there.

II. Insulin actually PREVENTS FAT BURNING. It causes your body to burn primarily sugar as its source of energy rather than fat.

III. Insulin is the hunger hormone. When it lowers blood sugar it often goes too low, setting you up for a cycle of craving and eating high-starch foods and too much of it, resulting in another cycle.

This is the Cycle of Obesity:
High blood sugar → insulin → low blood sugar → overeating → high blood sugar

This is not a game! If you are in this cycle you are at least pre-diabetic.

You can lose your legs, your kidneys, your eyesight, your life

An unfortunate fact:
Most overweight people are insulin resistant, meaning that because they eat too much Sugar and Starch, their muscle, fat, and liver cells do not use insulin properly. The pancreas just produces more and more, and excess glucose and insulin builds up in the bloodstream.

This is the scenario that produces obesity and _full blown Type 2 Diabetes_.

Insulin resistance makes losing weight incredibly difficult, and is VERY dangerous to your health.

This is not a game!

80 percent of diabetics are insulin resistant

2,200 people a day are newly diagnosed with diabetes

Diabetes is the 7th leading cause of the death in the United States

Diabetes is the leading cause of leg and foot amputations in the United States, leading to 86,000 amputations a year.

After an amputation roughly half of those people die within 5 years.

Heart disease is 2 to 4 times more likely with diabetes

75 percent of people who die from diabetes also have heart disease

Diabetes is the leading cause of kidney disease

Diabetes is the leading cause of new cases of blindness, up to 24,000 people a year lose their sight because of diabetes.

AND THE GOOD NEWS IS....

To fight being overweight, becoming insulin resistant, pre diabetic or acquiring Type 2 Diabetes you can follow **JJ's Way** and REVERSE this harmful cycle of obesity!

When you control insulin, you open the doors of the cells and allow the body to release fat. Glucagon to the rescue!

What do you need to do to lose weight and stop Type 2 Diabetes in its tracks?

It's quite simple:

EAT MORE

It may sound backwards, but it's true. You must EAT MORE to LOSE WEIGHT.

You need to eat more good food, more often. This is why in a Low Sugars and Starch Diet you will not get hungry between meals.

One of the underlying principles of JJ's Way is to not let yourself get hungry.

Not being hungry is the sign that your nutrition is properly fueling your metabolism.

Each day that you go without getting hungry
is a day that you are losing weight.

JJ's Way Eating Plan

The Eating Plan is a 3 Phase plan over the course of 12 weeks that will be integral to your 20+ pound weight loss. This is a high volume diet that will have you eating more often than you are typically accustomed to doing. Every 3-4 hours you will be eating measured amounts of proteins, vegetables, and in the later stages, unrefined carbohydrates.

The first phase is a 2-week initiation period where your body will get accustomed to the key principles of JJ's Way – switching the types of fuels your body uses and raising your metabolism.

The second phase takes place over an 8-week continuation period where your body is becoming accustomed to a raised level of metabolism.

The third phase is the last two weeks of the JJ's Way path to Discovery. By this time, you will have mastered the principles of eating frequently, eating foods that are largely unprocessed, fresh, and if possible organic, and you will have developed a keen ability to estimate portions, make good decisions about food substitutions and variations, eating out, etc. Most importantly, your body will have adapted physically to eating JJ's Way.

REMEMBER: The 12-week Eating Plan is not the way you have to eat for the long-term. The point is to master the principles and integrate these principles into a healthy lifestyle.

Getting Started on JJ's Way Eating Plan:

GROCERY SHOPPING LIST

PHASE I

◊ Eggs
◊ Smoked Salmon
◊ Grains – brown rice, whole wheat couscous, millet, quinoa
◊ Whole wheat pasta
◊ Plain yogurt (try Greek yogurt, it has much lower sugar content!)
◊ Vegetables – leafy greens (spinach, kale, collards), broccoli, asparagus, green peppers, cucumbers, tomatoes, carrots
◊ Chicken breast or skinless boneless thighs
◊ Flank Steak
◊ Any white fish (tilapia, sole, catfish)
◊ Salmon (try to find wild not farm-raised)
◊ Canned Tuna
◊ Canned Sardines
◊ Olive oil
◊ Cooking spray (Pam)
◊ Soy Sauce (low sodium)
◊ Dijon or spicy mustard (no sugar)
◊ Red Wine Vinegar
◊ Lemons
◊ Spices: Garlic salt, oregano, dill weed, basil, curry, paprika

PHASE II (includes all items from Phase I list)

◊ Fruits: apples, pears, all types of berries, pineapple
◊ Oatmeal or other grain cereal (no instant!)
◊ Whole wheat pita
◊ Legumes: Lentils (dry), garbanzo, black, Northern or pinto beans (dry or canned)
◊ Skim or low fat milk
◊ Cottage cheese (whole or low fat, no fat free, it typically has more sugar)
◊ Wheat or grain cereal (no sugar)
◊ Lean Deli meat such as roast turkey or beef

JJ's Way Phase I

The first phase is a 2-week initiation period where your body will get accustomed to the key principles of JJ's Way – *switching the types of fuels your body uses and raising your metabolism*.

This is a high volume diet that will probably have you eating more food - more often, that is - than you are accustomed to doing. Every 3-4 hours, you will be eating measured amounts of protein and vegetables.

Most recommended foods will be largely unprocessed, fresh, and if possible organic.

> *"In my first week of food shopping with the JJ's Way list, I saved $100 off my grocery bill."*
> *Dru B., JJ's Way JustBeFit Member*

THINK OF IT AS A 2-WEEK EXPERIMENT. Remember, this is not the way you will eat for the long term! This is short-term! You do not have to eat this way forever.

Calories will self regulate, don't be concerned. It is important to remember that Calories count, but Hormones count much more. At some point calories matter - like if you're taking in 3,000 or more a day - but by and large they don't.

Your body will take a few days to adapt to having eliminated Sugars and Starches on JJ's Way.

Drinking water is essential for fat loss. Without water the kidneys dump part of their burden onto the liver, which is the main fat-processing plant of the body. The liver then cannot metabolize as much fat. And in case you were wondering, the answer is "NO", diet soda is not the same as drinking water.

During this first phase, treat grains as if they are Sugar and Starch, they turn into sugar very quickly in your body, promote addictive eating habits, and trigger insulin release. Later once you have controlled insulin release in your body, you will be ready to work small amounts of whole unrefined grain and complex carbohydrates back into your diet.

---

3 BASIC RULES FOR PHASE I

**You will not only see immediate results
in how you look and feel,
it will give your body the "kick" you need
to continue making progress.**

1. NO REFINED SUGAR
2. No 'FAST' or 'JUNK' food.
3. No alcohol.

In general you can eat unlimited amounts of vegetables, and eliminate sugars, dairy, trans fats. You will increase your intake of good fats through olive or canola oil, nuts, and fish.

DETECTING REFINED SUGARS ON FOOD LABELS

Even if you don't eat sweets, the amount of refined sugar you may be consuming would surprise you. Over two-thirds of the refined sugar used in this country is added into processed foods. In other words, it's hidden in many of the things we buy at the grocery store. Even foods marketed as "healthy" such as granola, fruit bars, instant oatmeal, many sauces and marinades, etc. are loaded with sugar.

Even stuff that you wouldn't expect to have any sugar like breads, soups, cereals, cured meats, hot dogs, lunch meat, salad dressings, spaghetti sauce, crackers, mayonnaise, peanut butter, pickles, frozen pizza, canned fruits and vegetables, tomato juice, and a host of other products all contain sugar.

This doesn't even take into account the obvious sugary products like candies, cakes, ice cream, cookies, doughnuts, and soda pop.

The bottom line: The 'real' health food is the kind that you prepare and cook yourself from fresh, preferably organic, ingredients.

Phase I Plan

Gotta Eat A Breakfast – This is a "non-skippable" meal. Having a balanced meal before starting your day is crucial for kicking off your metabolism, providing energy, and preventing you from overeating at lunch. During this phase you will rely on protein as your primary energy source with little to no carbohydrates in for this meal. The key is to get into the habit of eating a breakfast. There's a reason why they say it's the "most important" meal of your day!

SELECT ONE OPTION:

◊ **Scrambled Eggs** – a protein packed meal and easy to make. Take out the yolks in 3 of the 4 eggs; I find that one yolk is enough to give it just enough flavor and color! Heat pan with cooking spray or 1 teaspoon of canola or olive oil. Add some diced onion, green pepper and/or mushrooms for variety, and scramble away!

◊ **Protein Shake** – 1 cup cold water, 4 TBSP of JJ's Whey Protein Powder (or equivalent serving size of commercial protein powder, make sure it's sugar free), you can also add a ½ cup of plain yogurt and some sweetener. Blend for 10 seconds on high.

◊ **Smoked Salmon (Lox)** – 5 ounces of this flavorful fish, serve with a few slices of tomatoes and/or cucumbers to balance out the flavor.

◊ **Turkey Sausage** – 4 ounces (usually 2 patties). You can heat up in the microwave or pan fry lightly with cooking spray. You can reduce this to one patty and serve with 2 scrambled egg whites for variety.

◊ **Yogurt and Nuts** – 1 cup of plain yogurt, you may add sweetener for flavor, top it with a heaping spoonful of your favorite chopped nuts (almonds, walnuts, pecans).

Remainder of the day: Eat small meals every 3-4 hours until bedtime – These are the remainder of your meals that you should eat every 3 hours up to approximately 1 hour before bedtime. If you are exercising make sure you have one meal about 30-60 minutes before the workout and one meal immediately after the workout.

CHOOSE ONE FROM EACH GROUP PER MEAL:

Protein	Carbohydrate	Vegetable
4 oz grilled or baked skinless chicken breast	1/2 cup cooked brown rice or wild rice	1 cup steamed broccoli, green beans, asparagus
5 oz grilled, baked or broiled whitefish, salmon or swordfish fillet	1/3 cup cooked whole wheat couscous ½ cup cooked barley, millet, or quinoa	1/2 cup cooked collard or mustard greens, kale, or spinach
5 oz cooked ground turkey or beef (90% lean or above)		1 cup raw baby spinach or arugula
5 oz sautéed shrimp or mussels		1 cup sliced steamed turnips
4 oz broiled boneless pork loin		3/4 cup raw baby carrots
6 oz canned tuna or sardines (packed in water or olive oil)		5 celery sticks
		½ of a cucumber, sliced

JJ'S WAY TIPS IN THE KITCHEN!

◊ Always have on hand a little olive oil, spices, garlic salt, pepper, and lemon.

◊ Make easy breakfast egg white omelets – keep in your fridge a few small containers with diced onions, green or red peppers, mushrooms, squash, chopped spinach, tomatoes, etc. Get creative and enjoy!

◊ When cooking rice or other grains, add a tablespoon of olive oil to water along with some spices, garlic salt, and pepper before bringing to boil. It comes out with much more flavor and compliments all different types of meat and fish!

◊ Pasta can be seasoned with drizzled olive oil and garlic salt and a splash of lemon.

◊ Steamed vegetables and greens salads can be drizzled with a little olive oil and lemon or vinegar. Dried dillweed also enhances the flavor of vegetables.

◊ Throw some grilled chicken over 2 cups of baby spinach, top with olive oil, lemon, salt pepper and dried dillweed, sprinkle with your favorite nuts (pine nuts are my favorite but almonds, walnuts or cashews are just as good) and you've got a delicious salad, you won't even miss the croutons!

Veering Off the Course

It is very natural that as an explorer you will veer off course.

Slip ups can happen...when you are practicing a new way of being, old behaviors sometimes hold on. Just because you experience a slip, doesn't mean you have to take a fall. If you eat something that is not on the JJ's Way meal plan, acknowledge it, then move on and keep following the program.

Thoughts such as "I really blew it", "Well I ate that, now I can eat this, too" or "I'll eat this and work out extra hard to work it off" are NOT consistent with your goals becoming healthier and leaner.

You don't have to continue to eat foods that aren't in your best interest. If you make the conscious, informed decision of eating foods with processed sugar, eat it slowly and experience it with your senses. Is this one of your favorite foods? If so, what about it do you like? What does the first mouthful taste like? What does it smell like? The texture?

Write down your observations in your Discovery Journal. By slowing down the process of unhealthy eating, you will likely find that you can have much less of foods that are sweet, and actually enjoy them twice as much. I am not encouraging you to deviate from your meal plan, but if you find yourself in this position, I want you to have the tools to better manage it.

Rate your hunger from 1 to 10 (1 being not hungry at all, 10 being so hungry you want to eat everything in sight). If you eat regularly, you will experience less uncomfortable hunger.

If you are uncomfortably hungry, you will likely eat more than you intended in a very short period of time.

If you are not physically hungry but ate anyway, what was the trigger for you to want to start eating? Stress? Boredom? Loneliness? It is important for you ask yourself these questions. If you can determine the trigger, you can come up with a different solution that does not involve stress related eating.

Each time you find yourself in this position, write your hunger number and a description of your situation in your Discovery Journal. The act of writing will help you understand and overcome your trigger. Be aware of every decision you make.

FYI – Cravings are mostly psychological. It may not feel that way, but they are. If you give them enough time, they will pass without a physical

> *"IT'S ALL ABOUT DECISIONS!"*

OFF COURSE CRAVER SAVERS

◊ *Celery / Carrot sticks*
◊ *Sugarless gum*
◊ *Flavored waters*
◊ *Diet sodas*

---

consequence. Cravings will at least decrease in intensity or even disappear in about 15 minutes. Although these can help in the short term, what sugarless gum and diet soda actually do is increase hunger, because your body expects there to be food to be coming because of the chewing/drinking. So it gets ready and then turns up the hunger volume because it has nothing to digest. A drop of honey on your tongue can act as emergency relief.

But let's keep things realistic and in perspective. If the choice is between a pint of ice cream or a pizza and a piece of sugarless gum or diet soda, NO DOUBT go for the sugarless gum and diet soda!

90% of the money spent on food in this country is on PROCESSED FOOD.

It's time to spend a little time in the kitchen. Try making your own food. It is a challenge and a learning experience, but it certainly beats your current experience of being overweight, tired, and depressed.

JJ's Way Phase II

The second phase is an 8-week continuation period where your body will get accustomed to the key principles of JJ's Way – *raising your metabolism*.

Like in Phase I, this is a high volume diet that will have you eating more food - more often – this is the key to effective weight loss. The difference between Phase I and Phase II is that you can begin working in more variety, including fruit, limited amounts of dairy if desired, a wider range of carbohydrate options.

THIS IS AN 8 WEEK EXPERIMENT – repeat this often to yourself over the next period to lessen the difficulty of change.

Don't forget the 3 Basic Rules, they still apply!

---

3 BASIC RULES FOR PHASE II

You will not only see immediate results in how you look and feel, it will give your body the "kick" you need to continue making progress.

4. NO REFINED SUGAR
5. No 'FAST' or 'JUNK' food.
6. No alcohol.

In general you can eat unlimited amounts of vegetables, controlled amounts of dairy, and eliminate sugars and trans fats. You will increase your intake of good fats through olive or canola oil, nuts, and fish.

One of the delights of eating JJ's Way is the many potential side benefits! During Phase II, you may find that the chronic headaches, allergic symptoms, inflammations, and many aches and pains you've had for years completely disappear!

The first 2 phases of JJ's Way eliminates many of the foods that are triggers for your food sensitivities (usually Sugar and Starch, refined grains, and omega-6 refined vegetable oils)

Phase II Plan

Gotta Eat A Breakfast – Again, it's a "non-skippable" meal. Having a balanced meal before starting your day is crucial for kicking off your metabolism, providing energy, and preventing you from overeating at lunch. This time around you will add carbohydrates to your breakfast in the form of a cooked unrefined grain – oatmeal is most available, but you may also find other options such as millet, oat bran, or a mix of several grains. Your local grocery store or Whole Foods will have several delicious packaged varieties. You could also find some whole grain cereal – but watch out for the sugar! Make sure that any cereal you buy has less than 2 grams of sugar per serving.

Protein	Carbohydrate
Eggs – scrambled, hard boiled, or pan fried in non-stick skillet.	Oatmeal or other hot grain cereal: 1/4 cup (dry)
# egg whites: 3	OR
# whole eggs: 1	Wheat cereal: 1/2 cup (dry) with ½ cup of skim or 2% milk.
Yogurt Parfait (3/4 cup plain yogurt with 1 serving cut fruit and sprinkle of nuts)	Note: no sugar but may use sweetener such as Splenda or stevia.
Protein Smoothie (1/2 cup cold water, 4 TBSP of JJ's Whey Protein Powder (or equivalent serving size of commercial protein powder, make sure it's sugar free), ½ cup of plain yogurt, ½ cup frozen fruit. Blend for 10 seconds on high.)	
Cottage Cheese with fruit (3/4 cup cottage cheese, 1 serving of fruit)	

Meals 2 through 5 – These are the remainder of your meals that you should eat every 3 hours up to approximately 1 hour before bedtime. If you are exercising make sure you have one meal about 30-60 minutes before the workout and one meal immediately after the workout.

CHOOSE ONE FROM EACH GROUP PER MEAL:

Protein	Carbohydrate	Vegetable
4 oz grilled or baked skinless chicken breast	1/2 cup cooked brown rice or wild rice	1 cup steamed broccoli, green beans, asparagus
5 oz grilled, baked or broiled whitefish, salmon or swordfish fillet	1/3 cups cooked couscous 4 oz baked potato or sweet potato	1/2 cup cooked collard or mustard greens, kale, or spinach 1 cup raw baby spinach or arugula
5 oz cooked ground turkey or beef (90% lean or above)	2 oz (uncooked) whole wheat pasta	1 cup sliced steamed turnips
5 oz sautéed shrimp or mussels	1 slice of whole grain bread or whole wheat pita	3/4 cup raw baby carrots
4 oz broiled boneless pork loin	1 whole grain tortilla	5 celery sticks
6 oz canned tuna or sardines (packed in water or olive oil)		½ of a cucumber, sliced

Variations that can be incorporated into Phase II:

◊ Add ½ cup of cottage cheese to your tuna, reduce the amount of tuna to 4 oz serving.

◊ Make turkey patties out of ground turkey, mix in some dried sage, grill or panfry and melt a thin slice of cheese on top.

◊ Add 1/8 cup of shelled sunflower or pumpkin seeds to your salads.

◊ Replace 2 oz of meat with ¼ cup of cooked legumes such as lentils, garbanzos, or black beans. Legumes are high in fiber and a great healthy alternative to meat. Season with some olive oil, salt, lemon, and parsley. I like to mix these in with salads or pasta.

◊ Deli meat can replace your grilled chicken or fish. Ounce for ounce. However remember that deli meat is often high in sodium and is processed so don't make it a habit.

◊ Add a tablespoon of natural peanut butter to your celery or carrot sticks. Peanut butter is also a great source of fiber and healthy fats!

◊ Fruit: Make sure that fruit is never overripe, as the sugar content is too high. That being said, it's now time to work back in some apples, oranges, and berries. Limit the sweeter fruits like bananas and grapes to a minimum. You can replace one vegetable serving with a piece of fruit (1 cup of cut fruit). But again, eat fruit in moderation (limit to 1 or 2 servings a day) for Phase II, as you don't want to risk causing spikes in your blood sugar.

◊ Throw some crumbled feta, bleu or goat cheese over your salads. Don't overdo it, remember the idea is to keep things simple!

JJ's Way Phase III Eating Plan

Phase III is a chance for you to loosen up on the rigid timing and food choice of Phases I and II of JJ's Way Eating Plan.

It is time to begin the practice of **intuitive living** by applying it to how you eat.

It is NOT the time to go "hog wild" and return to the Red Pill way of life. We've worked hard to speed up your metabolism and convert your body into a fat burning machine, let's keep the momentum going.

Remember, your destination is only a few weeks away.

During Phase III, you can be a little less strict about time between meals, but still very watchful about not getting hungry. You can also start estimating some of your portions. Don't worry, your body will tell you right away if you are under or over eating. Listen to your body!

Phase III is a great time to try dining out. Many restaurants have healthy menu options, and will often special prepare items without sauces that are high in sugar and salt. Know that oftentimes restaurants serve portions that are well over what your body needs and most people end up overeating. Our society is built around the idea of over-consumption: have the courage to be different! You're now trained to gauge the appropriate amount of protein, carbs and vegetables your body needs. Apply what you've learned at the restaurant!

Remember the 20 Minute Rule. It takes your body 20 minutes to register that it's full, so when in doubt eat less rather than more, wait awhile, then if you're still hungry have a bit more.

JJ's Way still encourages you to spend as much time in your kitchen as possible. Time to try all those healthy recipes! More JJ's Way recipes can be found at www.jjfitness.net/blog

Probably the best indicator that you're still on course during Phase III is the scale. During your weekly weigh in, if you notice that you are not dropping that pound or two a week (or more) that you have been, it is time to ease back and return to Phase II or even Phase I for a short period.

Chapter 8: Training

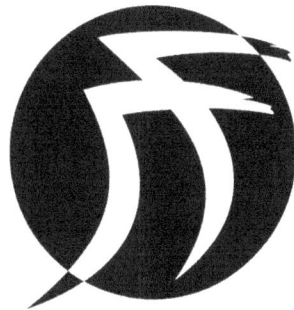

All explorers must plan a route and have a strategy. The JJ's Way Eating Plan is like charting your route. Training JJ's Way is the strategy to get to your destination.

The First Step of JJ's Way to Fitness is the Conditioning Phase. Later on you can focus on getting better at the movements and developing strength power and endurance.

This book deals with the First Phase of Fitness. During the last 4 weeks, you will likely begin the Second Phase, working on becoming more efficient and refining your technique.

There are 2 body states in the Conditioning Phase:

1. Deconditioned: an initial state of inactivity that is quickly changed
2. Conditioned: the natural state of the body and mind

In order to manage weight, the body needs to be in a conditioned state.

During the first 4-6 weeks of training JJ's Way, you will become conditioned.

While getting conditioned you will see and experience great change in body and mind – you will look leaner, stronger and toned, and you'll feel better and be more optimistic.

This initial conditioning phase training is about one thing:

Consistency

It is not about how long you exercise, how much weight you lift, or what incline the treadmill is on.

It's not even about how many calories you burn!

Losing weight is all about developing the **regular habit of exercise**!

In JJ's Way we will begin conditioning gradually.

You will not be spending hours of agony on the treadmill or bench pressing a truck.

We want to build slowly. Don't worry, you're still going to lose a lot of weight and get a lot stronger!

> ### JJ'S WAY HAS A FAVORITE SAYING ABOUT TRAINING:
>
> ### "IT'S A PROCESS!"

We do not encourage or expect rapid weight loss. "Fast food fitness" leads to gaining it and losing it, which is something that you've probably gone through many times already.

We practice a lifestyle of health and fitness. Weight loss is not slow by any means, but it shouldn't be on overdrive either! Resist the common tendency to be in a hurry to lose weight. Fitness and wellness is a continuum. Practice patience.

Start with the right mindset
Optimism and mindfulness are the keys to success in weight loss.

Like the body, the brain is very adaptable.

The brain 'listens' to every thought and records every move, adapting and setting patterns constantly. For example, many beginning trainees tell me as soon as we start, 'I am really uncoordinated.' This is a pattern they have set up for themselves, a mindset that the brain and the mind (two very different things) reinforces every time it's uttered, and carried through to the body in movement that results in either success or difficulty.

This is why I often tell someone who is entering into a balance move 'stop thinking and just do it.'

Optimism is one of the most essential parts of good training.

Optimism is a habit, an attitude of the mind

During this time of conditioning and initial weight loss, we need work on further developing three important lifestyle traits.

We call these the **JJ's Way 3 Qualities of Training**

The **3 Qualities** are:

1. **Consistency**: the regular habit of exercise

2. **Focus**: optimism, concentration and mindfulness during exercise

3. **Patience**: It's a Process. Enjoy the Process!

The 3 Qualities promote balance and wellness. The more that you can remind yourself of the 3 Qualities, the more healthy and balanced you'll feel. By repeating them to yourself throughout the day and during your training, they will develop within you and become a part of your newfound fitness lifestyle.

Warming Up

We always want to give your body some time to adapt to intense movement. This not only prevents injury, it enhances performance. You will work out better when you warm up. During Warm up your:

> Heart Rate increases
> Breathing accelerates
> Muscle temperature rises

The easiest way to warm up is to walk slowly – very slowly – on the treadmill. Resist the temptation to start to fast!

Several sets of jumping jacks, high stepping in place, side shuffles, or partial stationary lunges are also good options for a warm up.

Cooling Down

Cooling Down is one of the most important parts of working out. Don't cut your workout short by not cooling down!

If you are crunched for time, it is better to leave a set or two out of the workout than to not cool down.

Cooling down allows your body to return to regular temperature and the lactic acid (the stuff that makes your muscles burn when you work out) to begin to clear from the muscles.

Next day muscle soreness will be greatly decreased if you can remember to always cool down.

The best way to cool down is another very slow walk on the treadmill or pedal on the bike for five minutes.

Stretching

Most stretching should be done after the workout. These are the traditional stretches called static (non-moving) stretches. Use your stretch time for affirmation: you have finished your workout, and are taking an important step toward your health, your fitness, and your goals. Say positive things to yourself like "I did the right thing today" and "I met the challenge" or "I am becoming really good at the chest press".

Free yourself from any limiting beliefs and critical thoughts – these limit you. Repetition of personal and positive words is the key to reaching your potential.

"I am following JJ's Way and will lose my first 20 pounds" is a perfect affirmation. Express your affirmations as a conviction and they will change your life!

Write down your favorite affirmations in your Discovery Journal. Look at them often and say them out loud. The first few times will feel little awkward, but keep doing it. See how it affects your mental state and how that in turn affects your quality of life.

I do not recommend any kind of static stretching before or during a workout. There is no long term benefit to flexibility until after a workout, and there is evidence it actually puts your working muscles to rest.

Dynamic stretches – like toe touches - are for waking up muscles, not increasing flexibility. Dynamic stretches should only be done after warming up as a part of your workout.

While static stretching, is important to breathe into your stretch. Take a bigger than normal breaths and feel the tension release in your muscles. Visualize the muscle that is being stretched lengthening and relaxing.

> ### *Think: Long and Strong!*

The basic post-workout static stretches follow.

Quad Stretch
◊ Lay on side
◊ Support head with hand
◊ Pull top foot back until light tension is felt in thigh
◊ Breathe
◊ Hold 20 seconds, switch sides

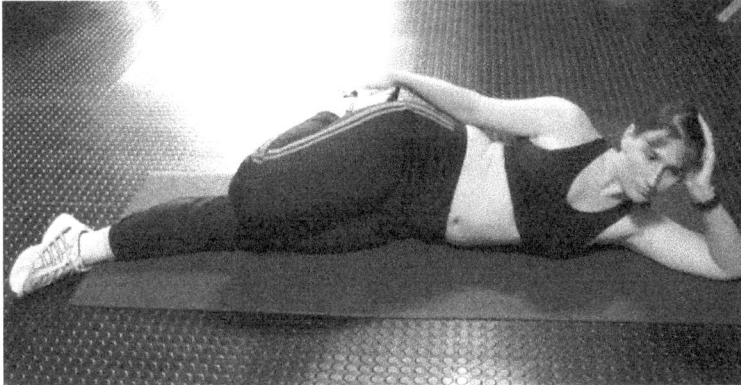

Hamstring Stretch
◊ Lay on back
◊ With a strap, belt or towel around foot, keep leg straight and pull gently
◊ Breathe
◊ Hold 20 seconds, switch sides

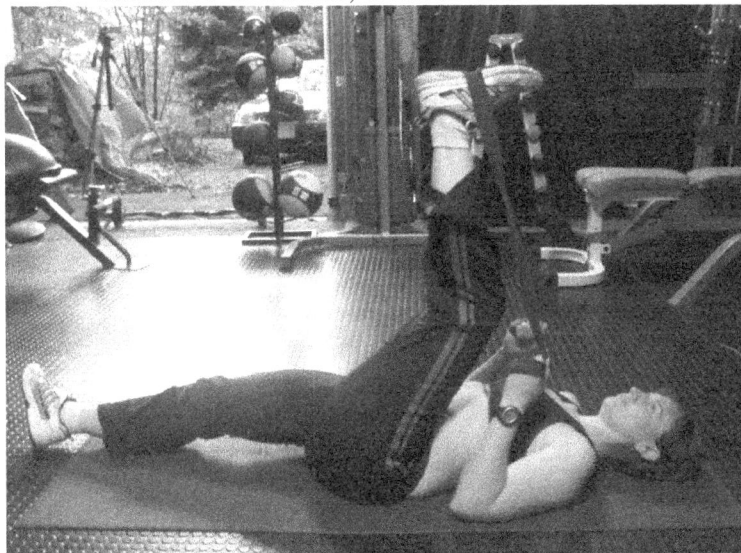

Glute Stretch
◊ Lay on back
◊ Pull knee to chest
◊ Breathe
◊ Hold 20 seconds, switch sides

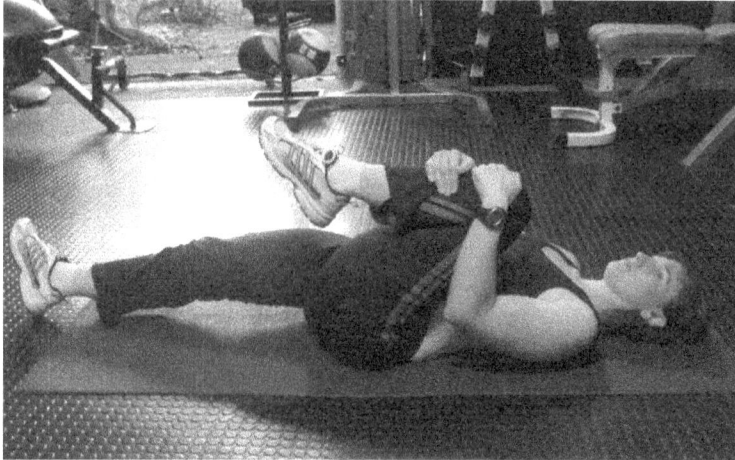

Outer Hip Stretch
◊ Lay on back
◊ With knee to side, pull lower leg towards chest
◊ Breathe
◊ Hold 20 seconds, switch sides

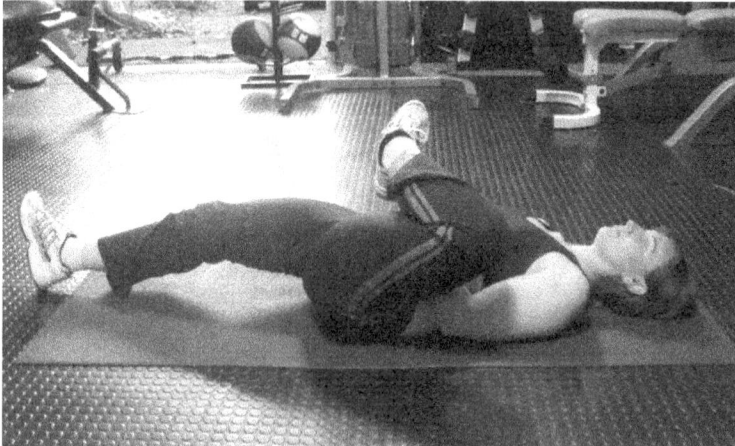

Lower Back Stretch

◊ Lay on back
◊ Pull both knees to chest
◊ Breathe
◊ Hold 20 seconds

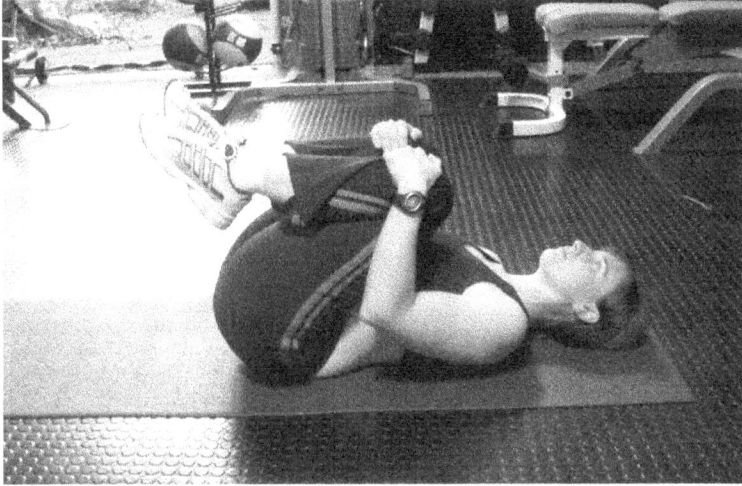

Chapter 9: Hara

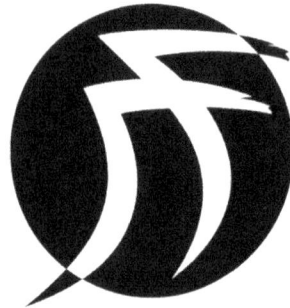

For thousands of years, philosophers have practiced the development of the trunk and torso.

The Hara, or as Core, is the physical center of our being.

Our sedentary lifestyle demands Hara training as a part of basic health.

I have saved scores of clients' untold amounts of pain and risk by steering them away from the doctor/surgeon path and into the gym.

80% percent of us, myself included, has experienced moderate to severe back pain. For that reason alone, Hara training is worth the small amount of time spent.

The Hara is a complicated structure, but by and large weakness, lack of flexibility and strength imbalance are more often than not the reasons for back pain.

GOOD NEWS: Because the Hara has the fastest growing muscles of the body, you can experience definite results in this area in 1-2 weeks!

Benefits of a developed Hara:
- ◊ Better posture and freedom of movement. (efficiency and relaxation)
- ◊ Improved muscular strength and endurance
- ◊ Improved power
- ◊ Improved motor control (athleticism)
- ◊ Decreased episodes of injury
- ◊ Improved flexibility

ALL movements either originate or are coupled through the Hara.

All force generated by upper and lower body musculature originates *in*, is stabilized *by*, and transferred *through* the Hara.

The muscles of the Hara:
> **Obliques** – the flanks. From your bottom rib to your hip on the sides of your torso. Controls side to side movement of the torso.
> **Rectus abdominis** – the six pack. From your sternum to your pubic bone in the front of your torso. Controls the tilt of your pelvis.
> **Transversus abdominis** – the main Hara muscle. Lays under the obliques and rectus abdominus and connects the front (rectus) to the back (erectors). Compresses the abdomen and controls forced breath.
> **Gluteus Maximus** – the buttocks, booty, butkus. Controls hip extension.
> **Hips (gluteus medius and minimus)** – the side of the glutes, lateral movement of the legs. Controls adduction of the legs.
> **Latissimus Dorsi** – a large back muscle that connects the ribs to the shoulder blades. Controls the shoulders
> **Serratus** – the muscles between the ribs. Supports the shoulder blades.
> **Rhomboids** – upper back muscles that contract the shoulder blades.
> **Erector spinae** – lower back muscles that keep the spine erect. Also flexes the spine.

As you can see from all the muscles of the Hara, static, one-plane strength training is inefficient, because the muscles of the Hara are capable of movements throughout a limitless number of planes.

If we train each part of the Hara in a variety of challenging ways, the whole becomes more powerful. This called **SYNERGY**.

The muscles of the Hara and back are interdependent.

A few guidelines for Hara training:
◊ Continue to breathe, and stay focused and relaxed through the entire set
◊ Stay slow and contracted
◊ As a trainee, your goal is to transfer the tremendous power potential of the Hara toward the working extremities without a loss of energy. This is done by maintaining good Hara position.
◊ Good Hara position: head level, shoulders down and back. Scoop the belly, pulling in and up.

Technique and Hara position are infinitely more important than additional reps and resistance. If you are balanced, you're Twice as Strong.

Remember: every rep of every Hara set - Perfect Form

Hara training is an important element of every JJ's Way Workout. As part of the Hara training, we do Focus exercises. Focus is a life technique to increase awareness, meditate on the body, and improve resistance training by raising consciousness.

The Focus exercises of JJ's Way are elegant, natural expressions of your self-growth. Although it may be tempting to hurry, take your time during the Focus exercises. Seek to get in touch with your Higher Self. Upon completion you will feel calm and of single purpose.

So far we've discovered:
Your magic number (anaerobic threshold),
your JJ's Way Eating Plan, and
your SYNERGY (Hara).

Now let's find out how you will be challenging yourself during your first month of working out with JJ's Way.

Chapter 10: Weeks 1 - 4 Training

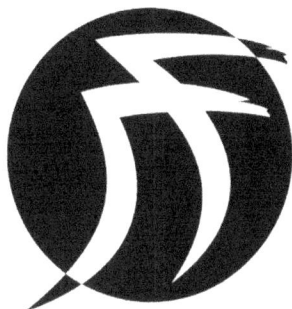

Now, the most exciting words in the English language: Let's Train!

I'm with you every step of the way. Remember, it's all about the simple act of doing. Just get started and let nature take its course.

After warming up, the first exercise will be a dynamic stretch and an exercise for the Hara. Next will be a superset of three exercises. Two for the shoulders, one for the legs. Supersets are a series of exercises during which you do one after another and don't take a break in between. The rest comes after you finish all three, then you do the series of three exercises again, rest, then one more time.

Supersets are challenging, and yet you can do it!

You will need to use as little, yes that's right, as little weight as possible to complete the supersets. Use just enough to make it tough around rep 12. As a rule, it is always better to use less weight than more.

After you have finished three sets of the first series, there is a second Hara exercise for your lower back.

Next, a shorter superset of two exercises, one for the shoulders, one for the lower legs. Do two sets of this series with a break in between.

A Hara exercise rounds out the resistance workout.
Finally, you do 20 minutes of Zone 2 cardio. **Your cardio workouts are on page 79.** Copy them into your Discovery Journal and record each workout.

There will be some exercises that you don't do well right away. That's alright! Like anything, it gets better with practice. Even after many years of training, I sometimes falter during a movement. No worries.

Keep it moving!

You might be inclined to think that some of the exercises are tough because you are out of shape. This is not always the case! Dips, Lunges, and Step Ups, for example, are hard even for the fittest of people. Hang in there and affirm yourself - Just Be Fit.

On the other hand, if something is too easy, you may be tempted to add more weight. Before you do, revisit the descriptions of form on the pages that follow and make sure you are doing the movement exactly right.

Finally, the pace of an exercise is very important. Be mindful that every movement has its own rhythm. Never hurry through a set.

Almost any exercise can be made easier by speeding up:

Slow Down And Let It Be Difficult

It's a Brave New World out there...time to discover it together.

Let's Train!

Indicates "Super Set"
Indicates "Hara" exercise

DAY ONE

PAGE	ACTIVITY	REPS	SETS	BREAK
67	Warm up	5 min	Zone 1	
81	Toe Touches	8	2	no break
83	Band Lateral Raise	12-15		
84	DB Military Press	12-15	3	90 sec
85	Band Stationary Lunge	12-15		
87	Hip Raise	15 sec	2	30 sec
89	Front Hold	20 sec	2	60 sec
90	Calf Raise	15		
91	Modified Leg Raise	10	2	20 sec
79	Cardio	20 min	Zone 2	
67	Cool down	5 min	Zone 1	
69	Stretch	5 min		

DAY TWO
Rest and Diet

DAY THREE

PAGE	ACTIVITY	REPS	SETS	BREAK
67	Warm up	5 min	Zone 1	
92	Side Bends	10 sec	3	no break
94	DB Chest Press	12-15		
96	Band Flye	12-15	3	90 - 20 sec
101	Band Squat	12-15		
103	Quad Extension	15 - 40 sec	2	30 - 10 sec
105	Band Curls	5 hold 10	2	60 - 10 sec
106	Push ups	6-8		
108	Crossovers	10 - 15 sec	2	20 - 5 sec
79	Cardio	20 min	Zone 2	
67	Cool down	5 min	Zone 1	
69	Stretch	5 min		

DAY FOUR

PAGE	ACTIVITY	REPS	SETS	BREAK
67	Warm up	5 min	Zone 1	
81	Toe Touches	8	2	no break
109	Band Low Row	12-15		
110	DB Pullover	12-15	3	90 - 20 sec
112	Step Up	24		
113	Bridge Track	8	2	30 Sec
114	Pulldown	12-15		
115	Single Leg Lateral Lift	10	2	60 - 10 sec
118	Frog Leg Crunch	10 - 15	2	20 - 5 sec
119	Sprinter stretch	20 sec	2	no break
	NO CARDIO!!!			
67	Cool down	5 min	Zone 1	
69	Stretch	8 min		

DAY FIVE

Rest and Diet

DAY SIX

PAGE	ACTIVITY	REPS	SETS	BREAK
67	Warm up	5 min	Zone 1	
121	Tip Toe Track	10	2	20 sec
122	Donkey Kick	12-15		
123	Dip	12-15	3	90 - 20 sec
125	Romanian DB Pull	12-15		
127	4 point balance	1 min	2	30 - 10 sec
128	DB Flye	12-15		
129	Band Leg Abduction	12-15	2	60 - 10 sec
130	Plank	15 - 45 sec	2	30 - 10 sec
131	Tree Pose	1 min	1	
79	Cardio	20 min	Interval	
67	Cool down	5 min	Zone 1	
69	Stretch	5 min		

DAY SEVEN

Rest and Diet

JJFitness Cardio
(Grab your magic number and Zones recorded on pg. 33 and fill in below!)

Zone 2 Workout
Highly Efficient Fat Burning
Builds Aerobic Base
Medium Intensity

	INCLINE	SPEED	HEART RATE	TIME
Warm Up	2.0	2.0 – 2.5	Zone 1:	5 min
Workout	2.0 – 6.0		High Zone 2:	20 min
Cool Down	2.0	2.5 – 2.0	Zone 1 (After 1:30):	5 min
TOTAL				**30 min**

Intervals Workout
Intense Fat Burning
Builds Aerobic Endurance
Medium/High Intensity

	INCLINE	SPEED	HEART RATE	TIME
Warm Up	2.0	2.0 – 2.5	Zone 1:	5 min
Ramp Up	2.0 – 6.0		Mid Zone 2:	2 min
Interval 1	4.0 – 8.0		Mid Zone 3:	2 min
Recovery 1	2.0 – 6.0		Mid Zone 2:	2 min
Interval 2	4.0 – 8.0		Mid Zone 3:	2 min
Recovery 2	2.0 – 6.0		Mid Zone 2:	2 min
Interval 3	4.0 – 8.0		Mid Zone 3:	3 min
Recovery 3	2.0 – 6.0		Mid/High Zone 2:	2 min
Interval 4	4.0 – 8.0		Mid Zone 3:	3 min
Recovery 4	2.0 – 6.0		Mid/High Zone 2:	2 min
Cool Down	2.0	2.5 – 2.0	Zone 1 (After 1:30)	5 min
TOTAL				**30 min**

Weeks 1 - 4 Exercises

As a discoverer you <u>must</u> stay aware and maintain focus. Don't back away from challenges. This is the opportunity of lifetime.

While you workout, let nothing distract you from your goal. Your goal is to lose that first 20 pounds and become fit and healthy.

For the first 2 weeks of any new workout, concentrate on getting the form of the exercises. The pace and tempo will follow naturally.

Be aware of your body, your mind, <u>and</u> your environment!

> *"DON'T FORGET TO BREATHE!"*

Look for opportunities to be optimistic!

Remember to have your Discovery Journal on hand, and a timing device (like your Heart Rate Monitor or a stopwatch) to keep track of intervals.

Hara: **Toe Touches**

◊ Stand with toes on 2-4 inch step, heels on ground
◊ Reach up with both hands and breathe in deeply
◊ Pull in Hara midsection
◊ Reach hands down in a circular motion and visualize reaching around a large beach ball while exhaling
◊ At the bottom, finish exhale, keep belly pulled up and in, and, keeping your arms around the beach ball, return to start position
◊ Do 8 reps and focus on breathing. Pace is medium, not slow

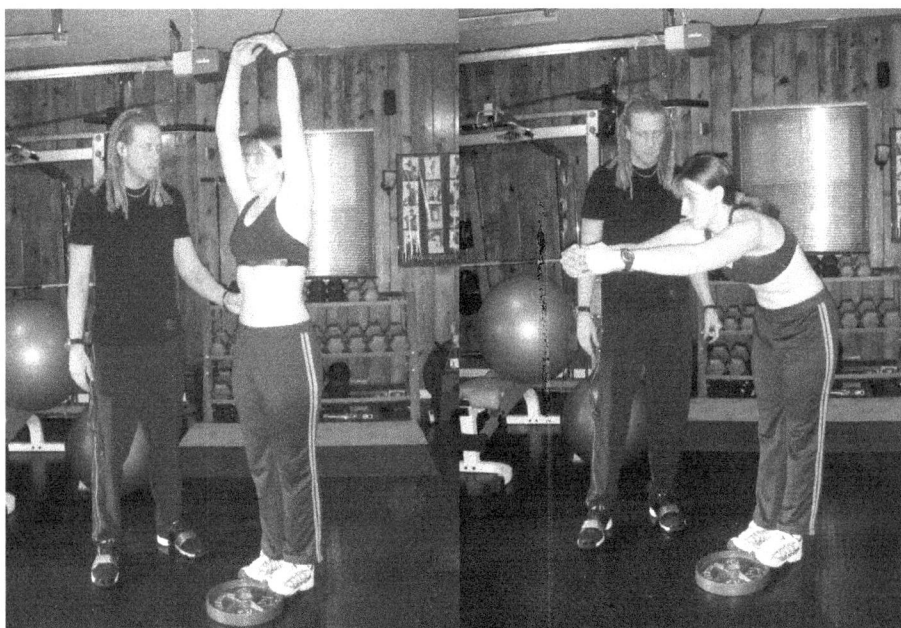

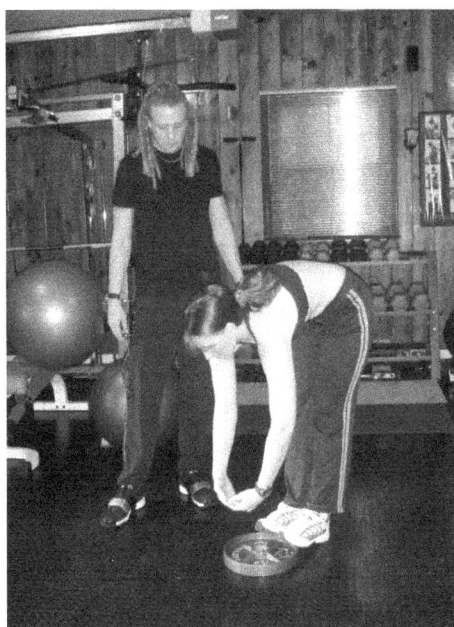

◊ Step over to stand with heels on same step, toes down
◊ Same as above. Do 8 reps with focus on breathing. Pace is medium, not slow

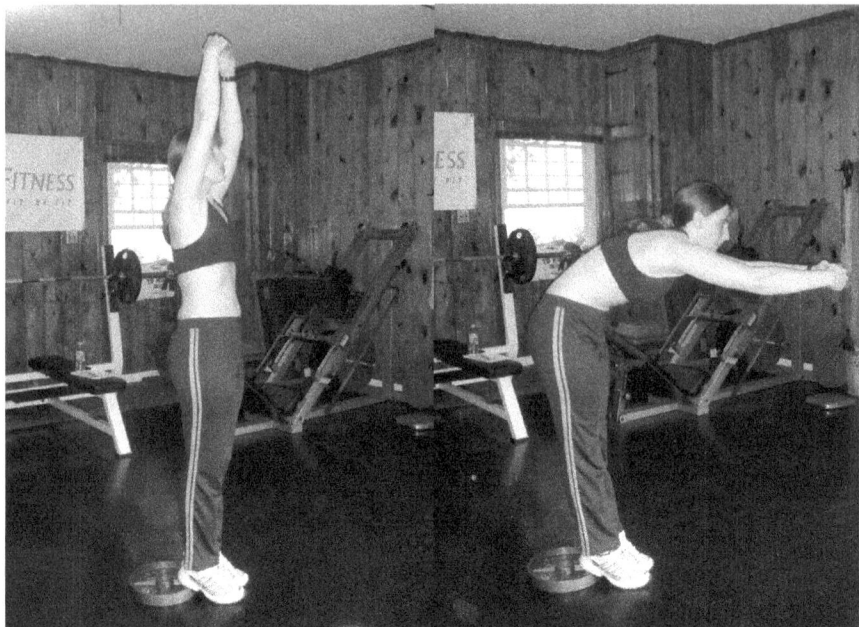

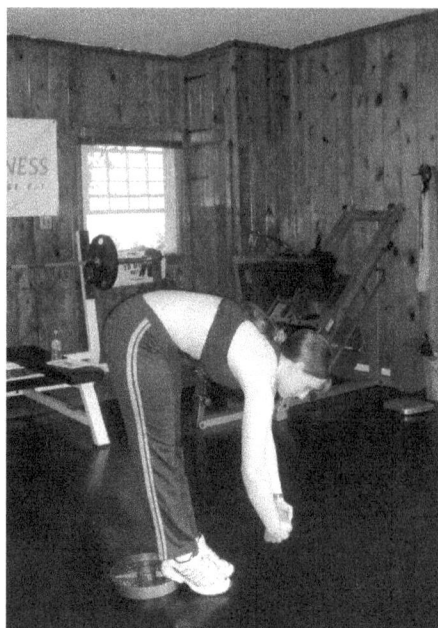

Shoulders: **Lateral Raise (Band or Dumbbell)**

◊   Stand with both feet on resistance band (or if using dumbbells less than shoulder length apart)
◊   Raise arms laterally. Keeps hands below shoulder level. Visualize that your arms are airplane wings
◊   At top position, pause a quarter beat. Keep hands below shoulder level
◊   Return slowly, feeling tension on band

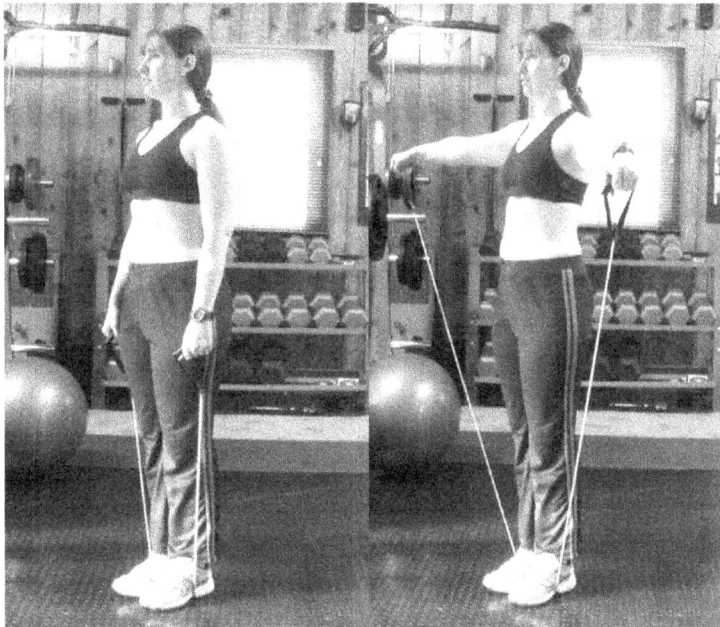

Shoulders: **Dumbbell Military Press**

◊ Sit in good Hara posture on Swiss Ball
◊ Raise dumbbells to position level with ears
◊ Press slowly, keep arms soft at top, bringing hands nearly together. Visualize how great your shoulders are going to look!
◊ Return slowly

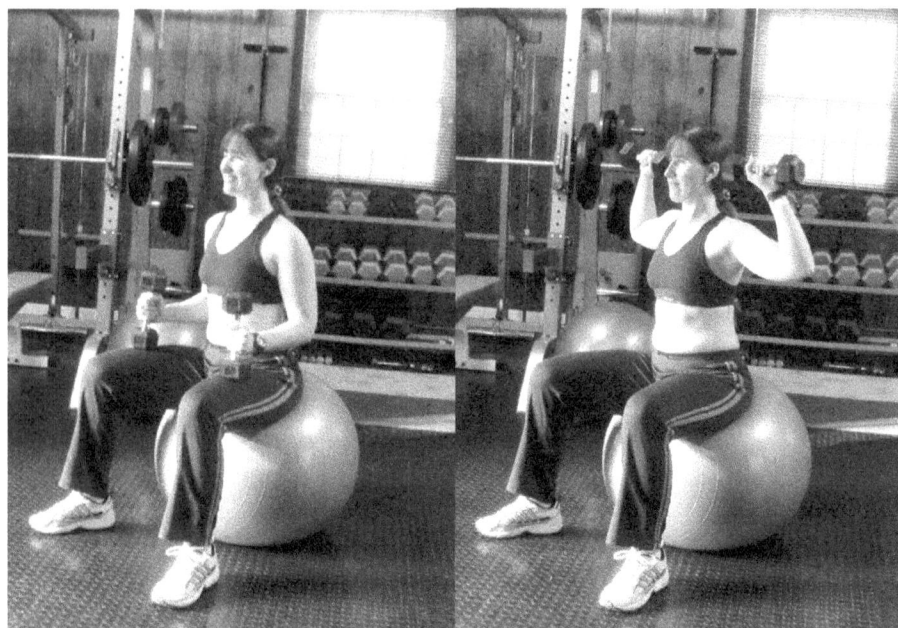

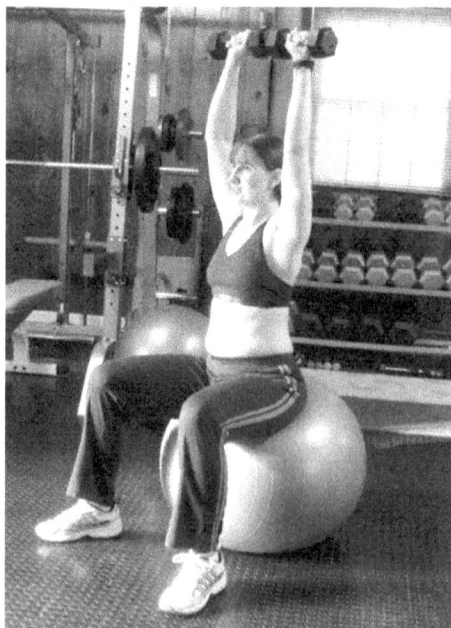

Quads, Hamstrings: **Band Stationary Lunge**

◊ Behind with band under one foot, band in both hands, hands at shoulder level
◊ Take a large step back, then another half step just out of comfort zone, staying balanced
◊ Back foot should be in line and on toes
◊ Establish good Hara tension, keep chin up and torso straight
◊ Lower till knee is almost touching the ground
◊ Make sure your knee of your front leg is behind your toes
◊ Press through the heel of the front foot up to starting position
◊ Do partials if necessary to build adequate strength
◊ When done properly, this is a very statuesque movement. Visualize that you are posing for a great sculptor

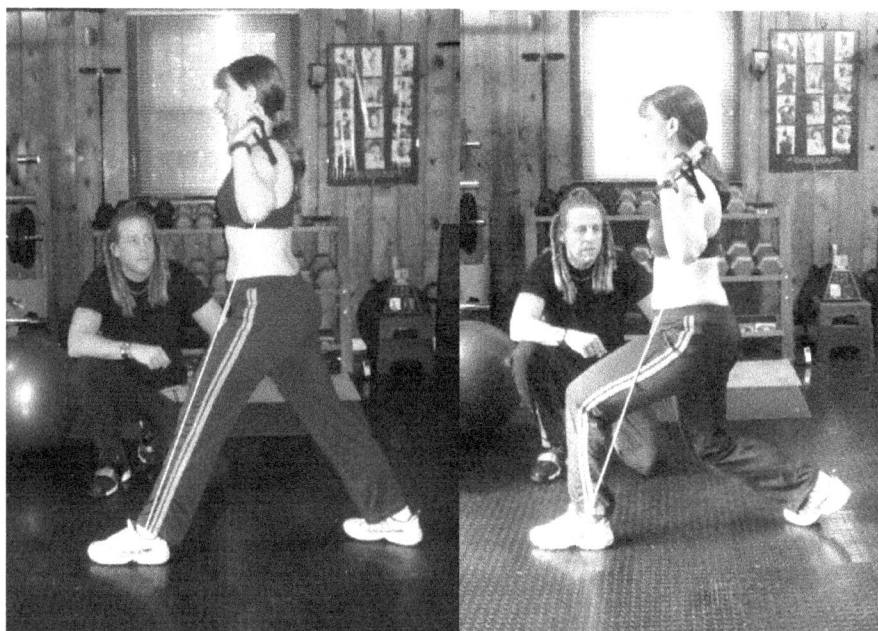

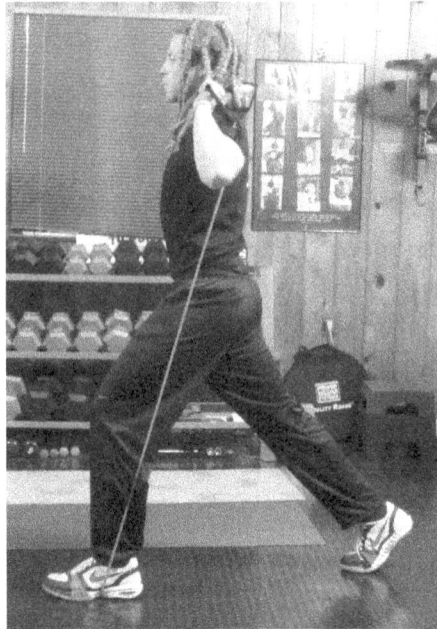

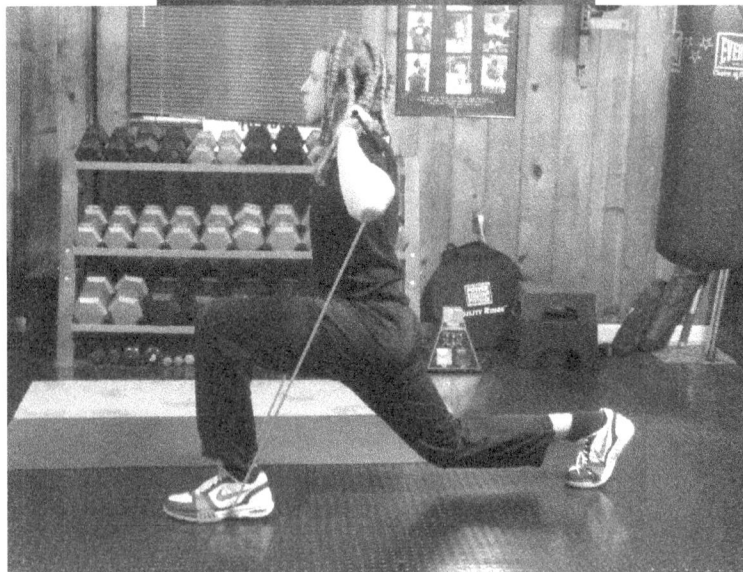

Hara: **Hip Raise**

◊ Lay flat on mat, knees bent, feet flat, hands to the side
◊ Raise hips to form a 'plank' from shoulders to knees
◊ Visualize that your body is a plank
◊ Hold for designated time, then lower slowly to rest

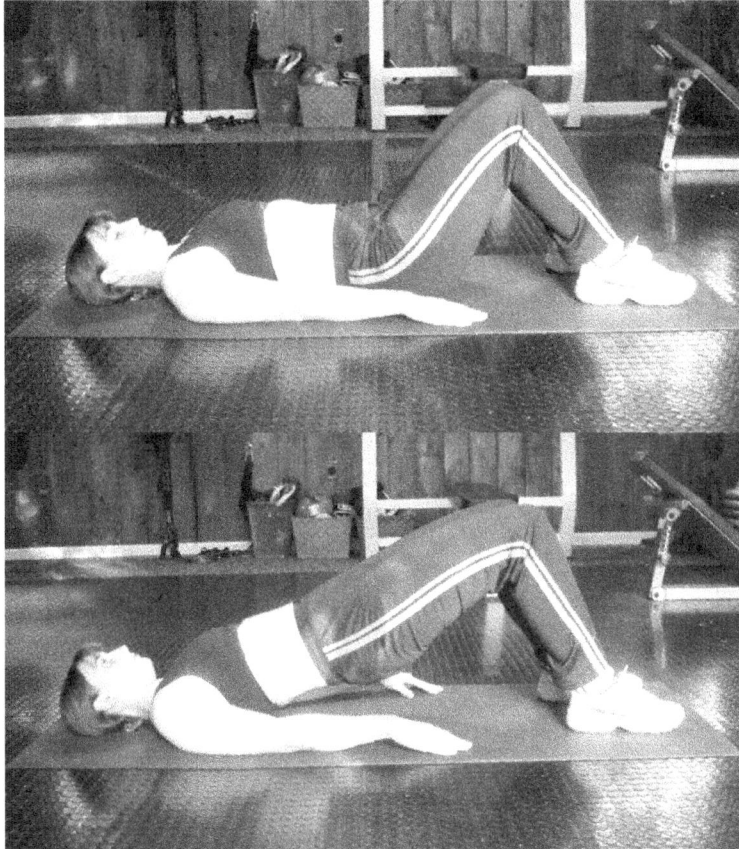

◊ Progress from feet on mat, to Bosu Disc, then Swiss ball as balance and strength allow

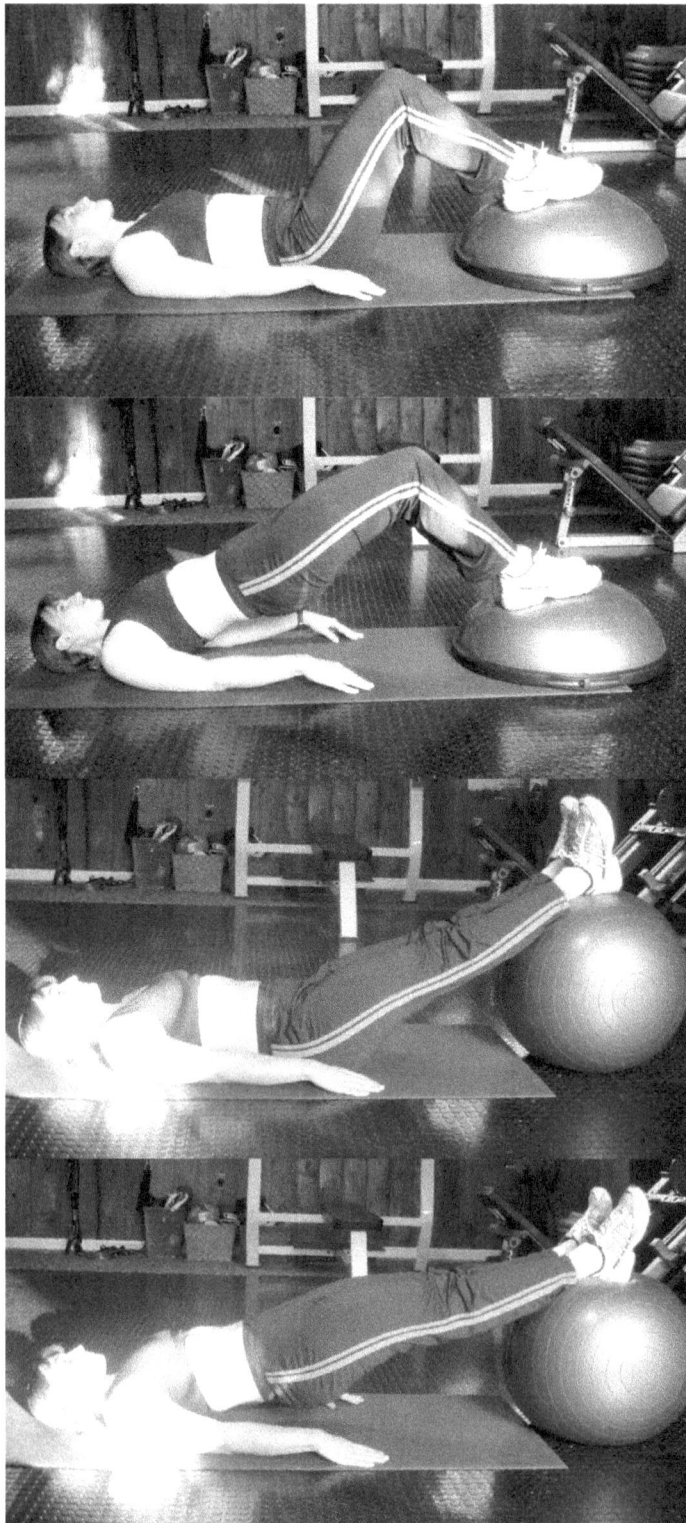

Shoulders: **Front Hold with Band**

◊ Stand with band under both feet, hand in front
◊ Establish good Hara position
◊ Raise hands to just below shoulder level
◊ Visualize that you are a monk of the Shaolin Temple, and this is your test of willpower and mental focus
◊ Hold until designated time, lower slowly
◊ You must consciously make and effort to maintain good Hara position throughout

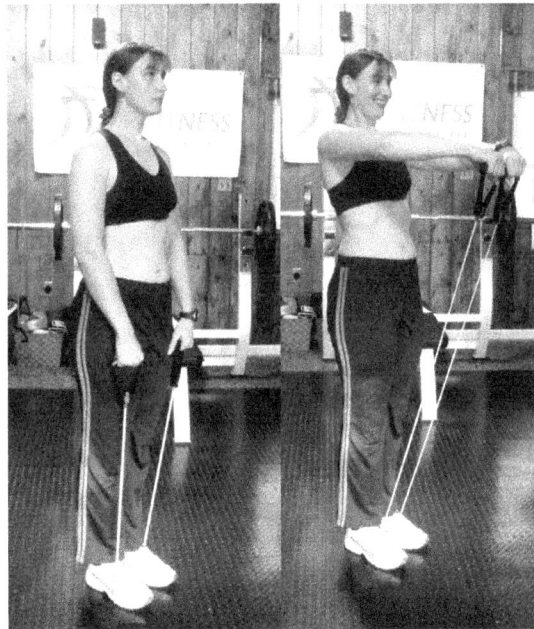

Calves: **Calf Raise**

◊ Stand with balls of feet on step or stair
◊ Use one hand to balance against a partner or stationary object
◊ Lower through full range of motion
◊ Raise to top of range of motion. Visualize that you are a dancer, with powerful, lively legs, and are preparing for a performance
◊ Slowly repeat
◊ You must consciously keep a slow and steady pace

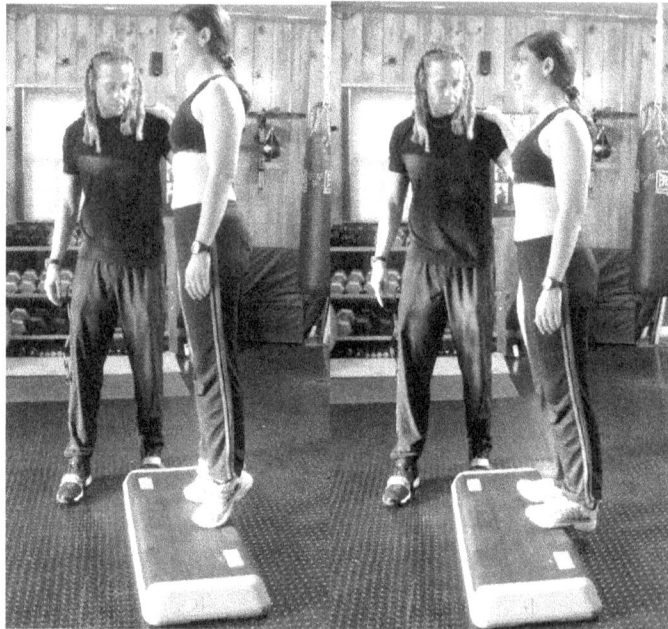

Hara: **Modified Leg Raise**

◊ Lay on back with knees bent
◊ Place hands halfway under hips and adjust so that lower back lays flat on ground
◊ Bring legs to 'table top' position
◊ Keeping legs at 90 degree angle, slowly lower feet to tap the mat
◊ Slowly return. Visualize that you are a builder laying a foundation for a strong building (your Hara)

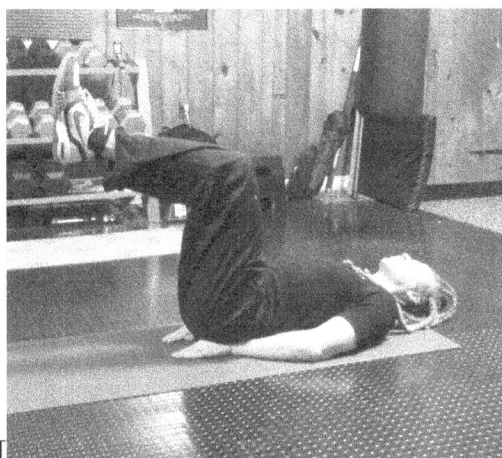

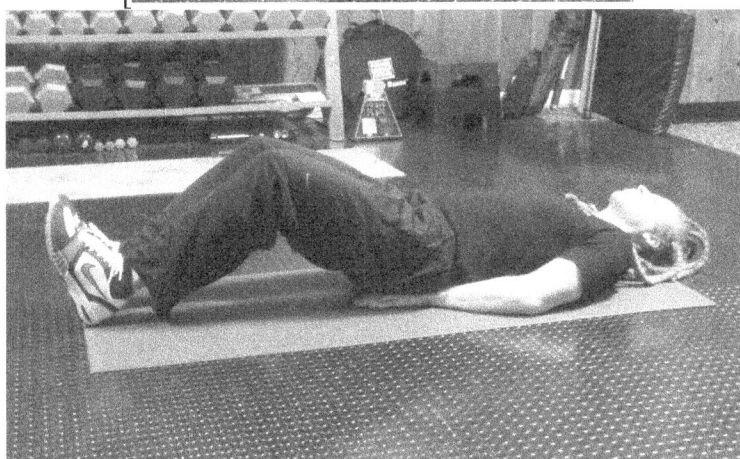

Hara: **Side Bends**

◊ Stand in good Hara position, hands on hips
◊ Using left hand as a support bend to the left
◊ Hold position for designated time, breathing throughout
◊ Return slowly and repeat to the right

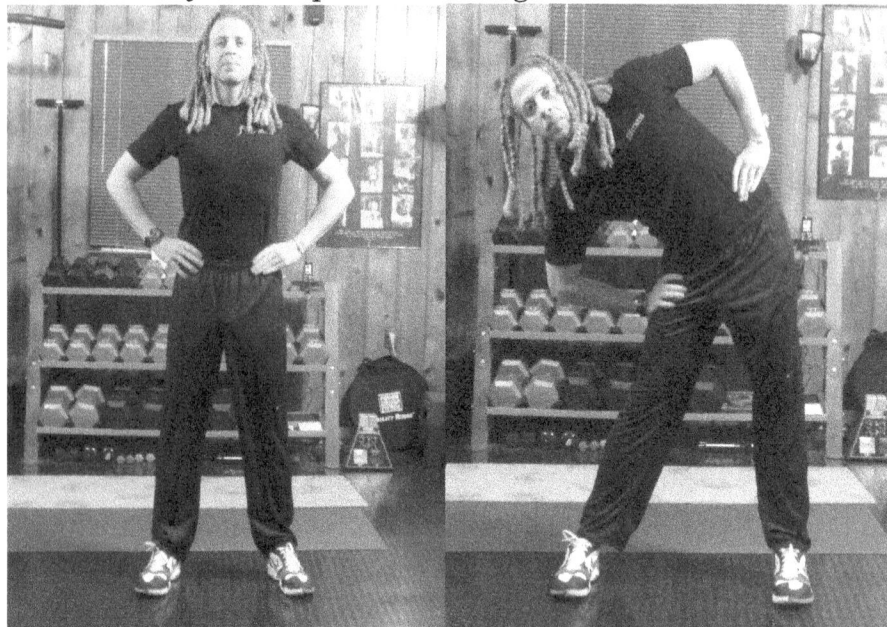

◊ For second set, progress by extending opposite arm over head, increasing required effort
◊ On final set remove support hand
◊ Visualize your oblique muscles getting Long and Strong!

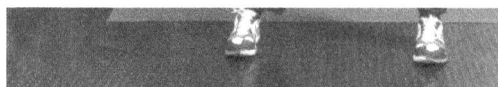

Hara: **Bridge on Swiss Ball**

◊ Sit in good Hara posture on Swiss Ball
◊ Roll forward until head and shoulders are on ball
◊ Neck must be relaxed
◊ Raise hips to form a 'plank' from shoulders to knees
◊ Visualize that you are a coffee table with delicate china sitting on your stomach
◊ Hold for designated time
◊ Using abdominal muscles, roll slowly back to sitting position

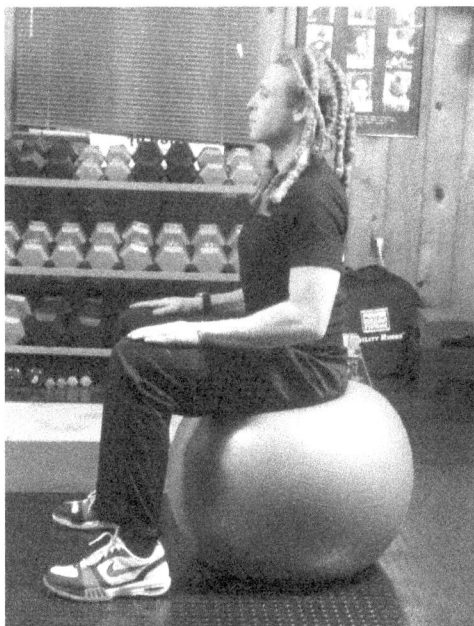

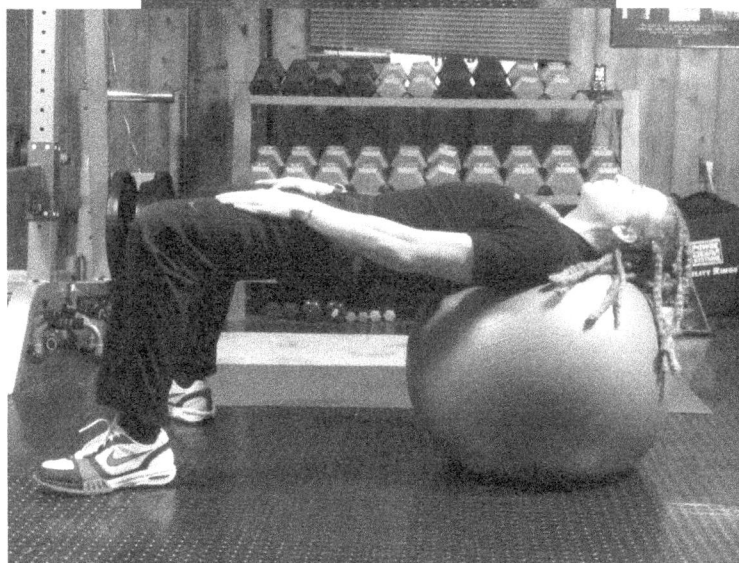

Chest: **Dumbbell Chest Press**

(Before starting, practice "Bridge on Swiss Ball" exercise on pg. 93 in preparation for Chest Press on ball)

◊ Start by sitting in good Hara posture on the Swiss Ball

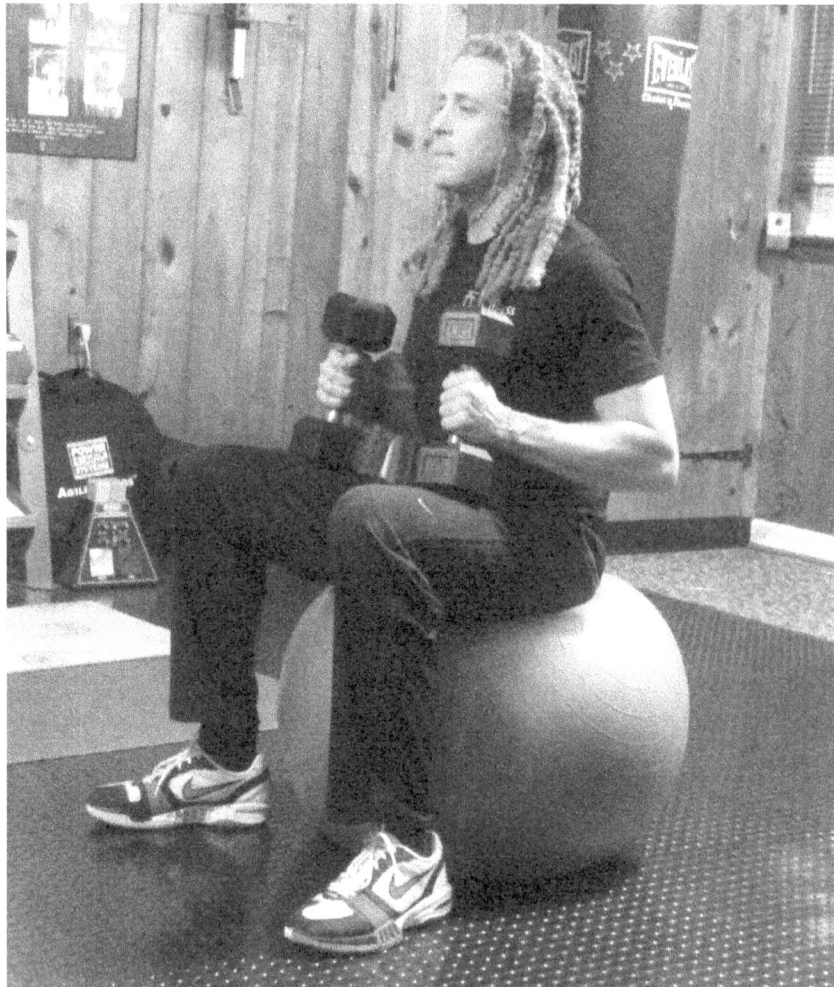

◊ Roll forward into a bridge position, keeping dumbbells resting on torso
◊ Rotate dumbbells to position even with lower chest
◊ Press slowly, keep arms soft at top, bringing hands nearly together. Visualize that you are pressing up to and through the ceiling
◊ Return slowly

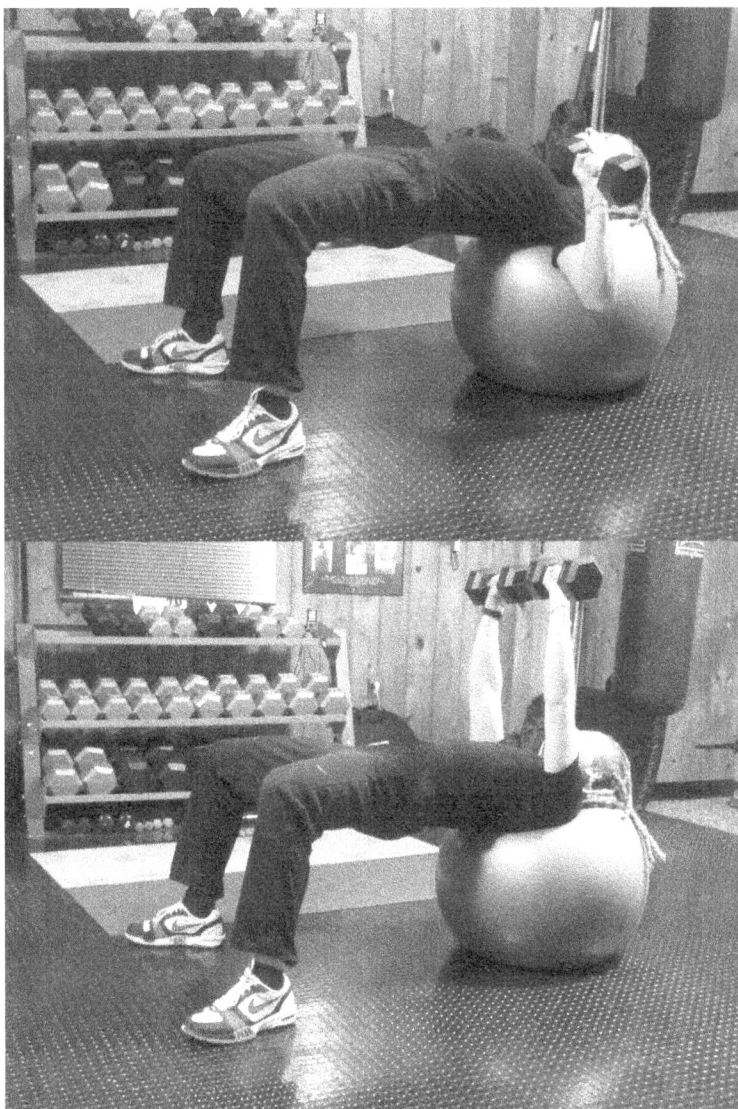

Chest: **Band Flye**

◊ Secure band to secure object behind and at shoulder level. Face away.
◊ Stand in stagger step.
◊ Take handles at shoulder height, palms facing arms long and slightly bent.
◊ Slowly spread arms until stretch is felt in chest. Keep arms 'soft' at 15 degrees.
◊ Visualize hugging a big bag of rice
◊ Slowly return, bringing palms together and flexing chest.

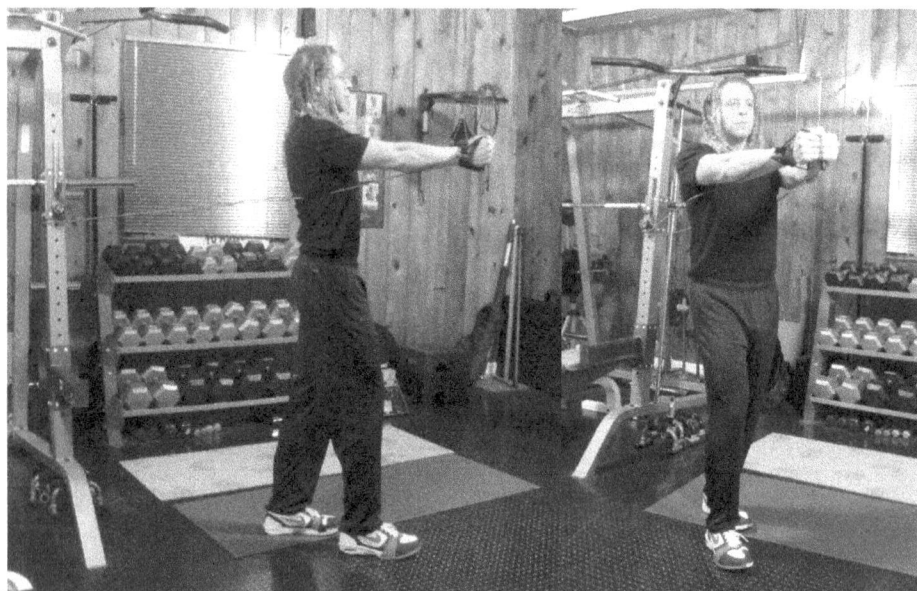

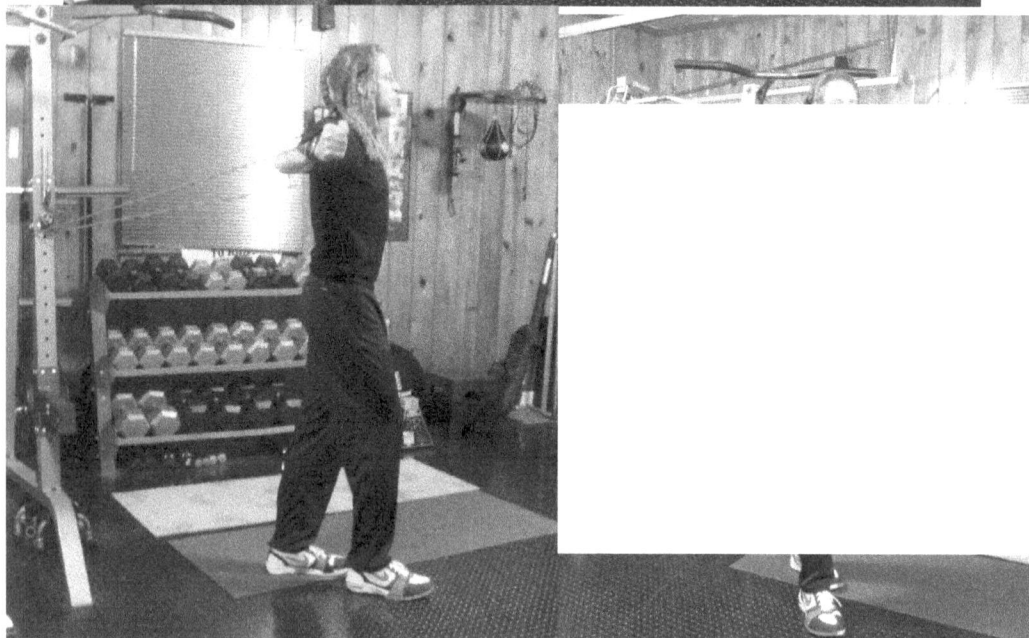

Quads, Hamstrings: **Squat with Bench** (preparing to squat)

◊ Sit on a chair or bench so that upper leg from knee to hip is roughly parallel to the ground.

◊ Position feet wider than shoulder width, flaring feet 5 degrees if comfortable.

◊ Hold arms straight in front (like Frankenstein)

◊ Lean torso forward

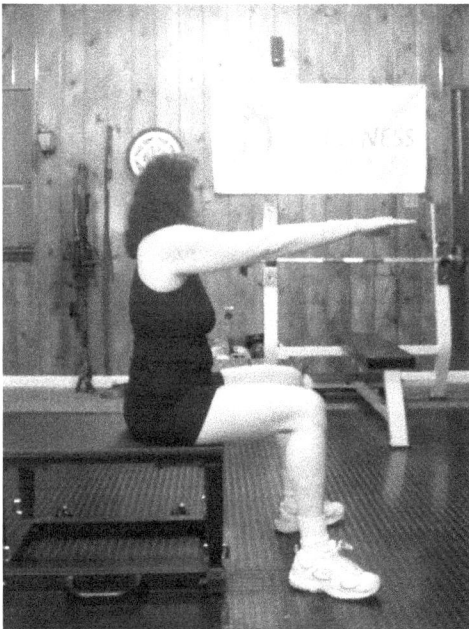 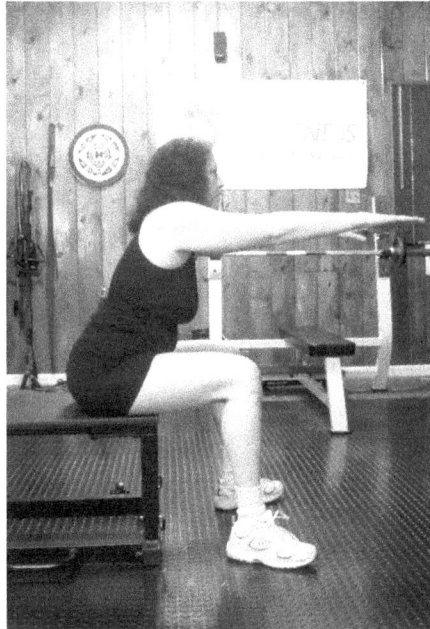

◊ Stand, press though heels (rear wheel drive) keep chin up and feet in place.
◊ Keeping legs straight and chin up, lean forward, bending at hips.
◊ Keeping knees behind toes and rear wheel drive in heels, slowly bend knees to sit
◊ The bench squat is a one part movement standing up, and a two part movement – hip bend before knee bend – sitting down

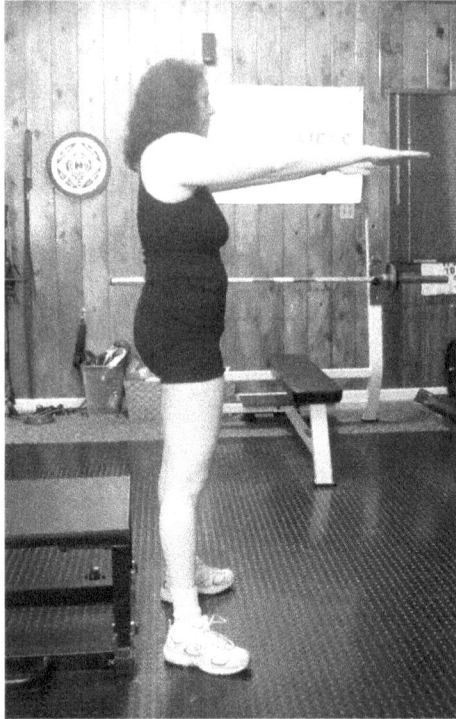

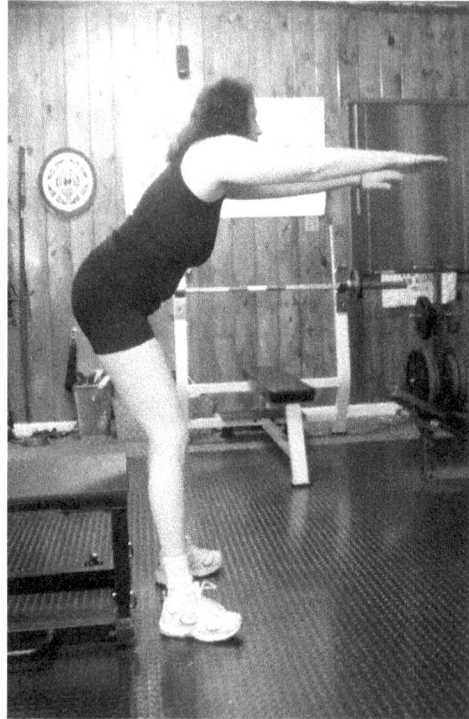

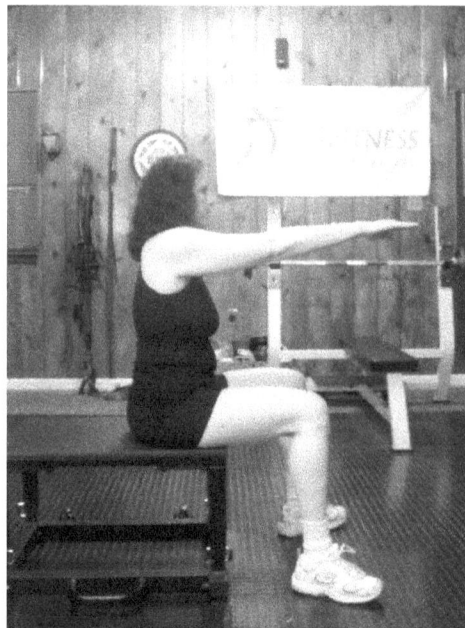

Quads, Hamstrings: **Partial Squats**

(Before starting, practice the "Squat with Bench" exercise on pg. 97-98 to prepare for a full squat)

◊ Remove bench
◊ While standing position feet wider than shoulder width, flaring feet 5 degrees if comfortable
◊ There is no universal foot position, but most people will want their feet wider rather than closer
◊ Hold arms straight in front (like Frankenstein)
◊ Lean torso forward, keeping legs straight and bend at hips. Hold chin up
◊ Keeping knees behind toes, bend knees to 45 degrees, pressing though heels (rear wheel drive) keep chin up and feet in place
◊ Press through rear wheel drive to standing position
◊ The squat is a two part movement going down – hip bend before knee bend – and a one part movement coming up

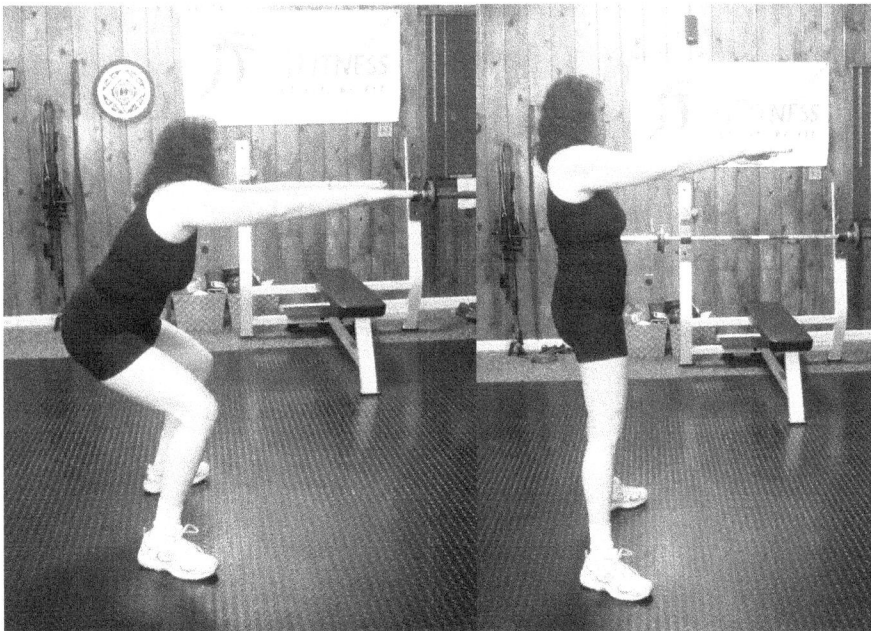

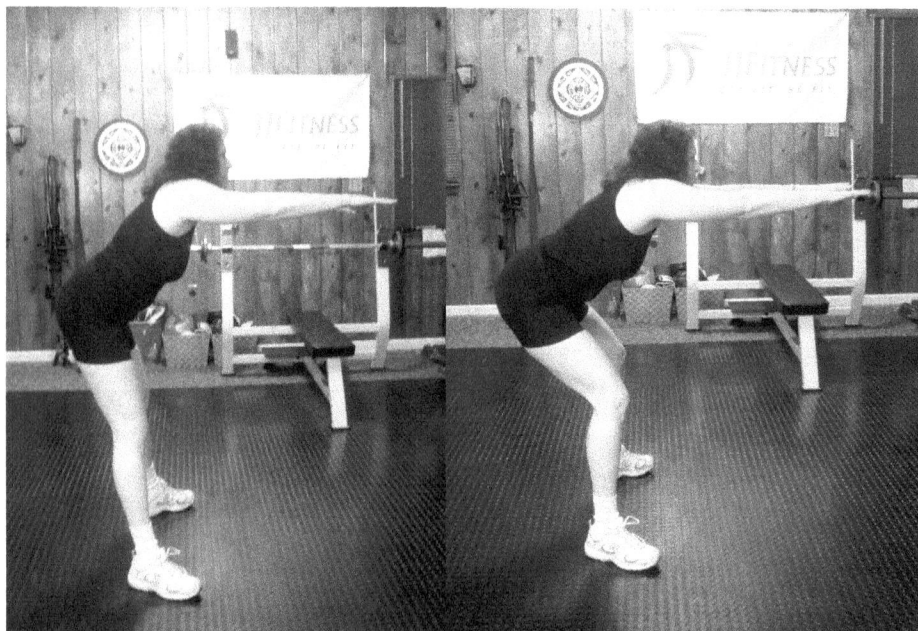

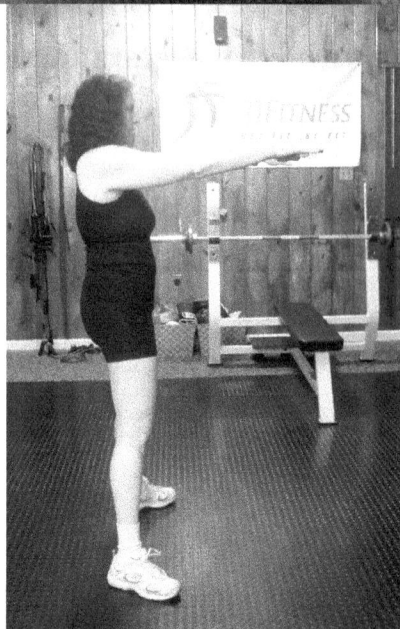

IMPORTANT NOTE ABOUT DOING SQUATS:

It may take you several weeks to "find your groove" when working on your squat. Focus on perfecting your form, don't worry about how hard or easy it feels.

Quads, Hamstrings: **Band Squats**

(Before starting, practice the "Squat with Bench" exercise on pg. 97-98 to prepare for a full squat)

◊ Stand on band with both feet
◊ While standing position feet wider than shoulder width, flaring feet 5 degrees if comfortable
◊ There is no universal foot position, but most people will want their feet wider rather than closer
◊ Rotate hands and bring them to shoulders
◊ Lean torso forward, keeping legs straight and bend at hips. Hold chin up
◊ Keeping knees behind toes, bend knees to 45 degrees, pressing though heels (rear wheel drive) keep chin up and feet in place
◊ Press through rear wheel drive to standing position
◊ The squat is a two part movement going down – hip bend before knee bend – and a one part movement coming up
◊ When you get strong enough to do a full deep knee bend squat, visualize a marble on your mid-thigh that does not roll forward or back

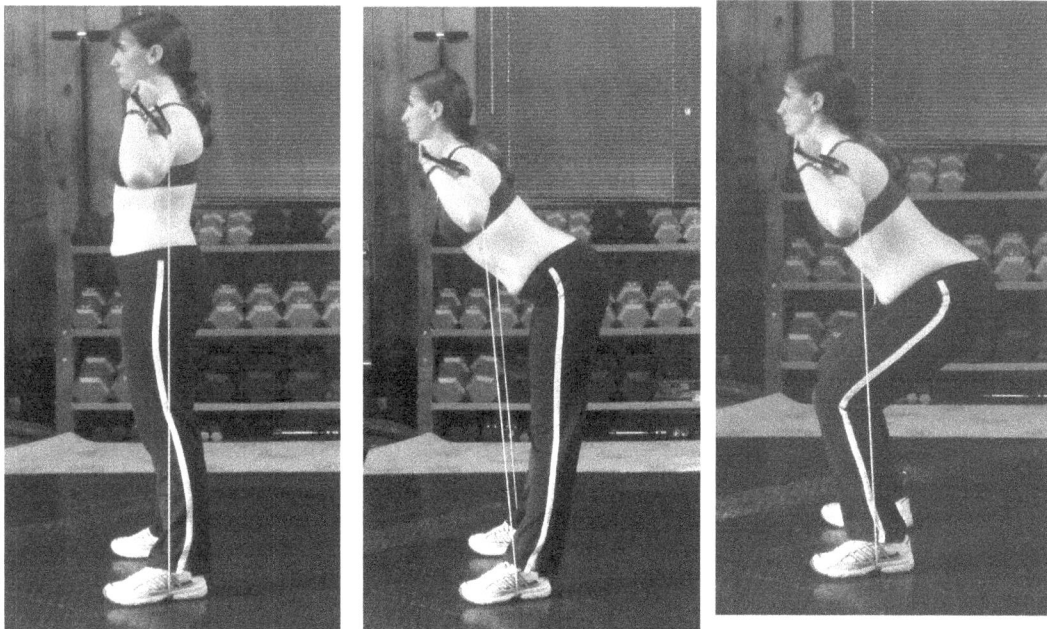

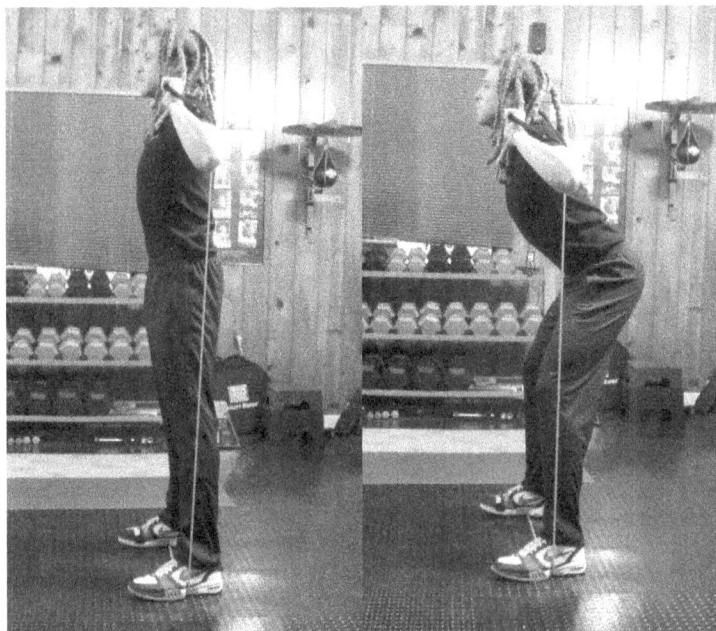

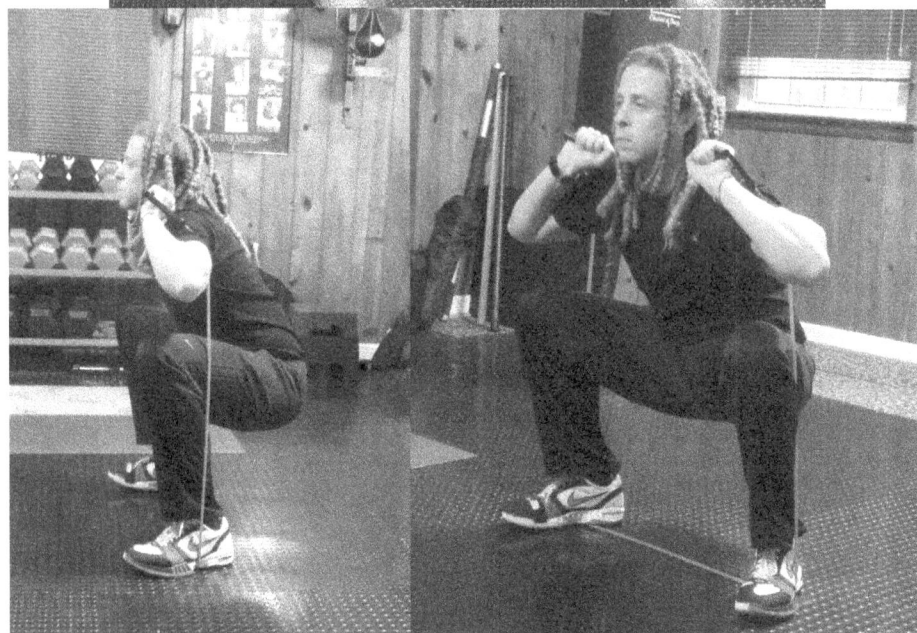

Hara: **Quad Extension**

◊ Establish good Hara position on hands and knees
◊ Keep head up
◊ Slowly extend right leg back and straight. Visualize that you are a circus performer and must balance a ball on your extended foot
◊ Hold position for required time
◊ Come back slowly to start position
◊ Switch legs

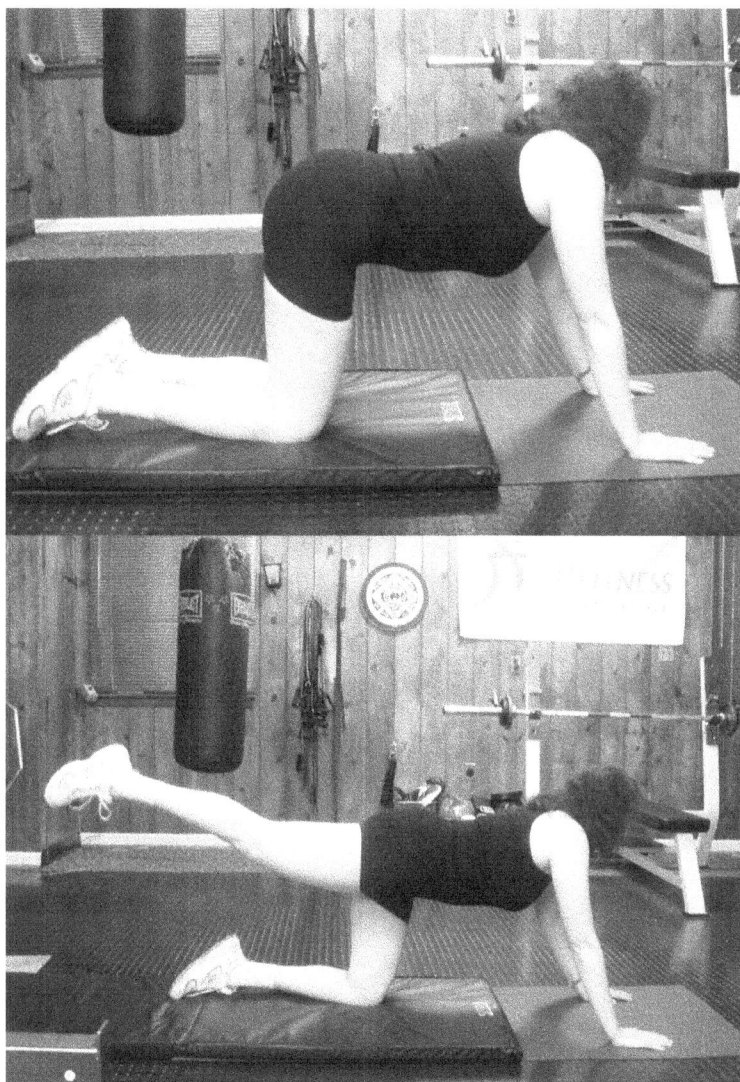

◊ To increase difficulty, extend opposite arm in hold position
◊ Visualize that you are a bird dog during duck season

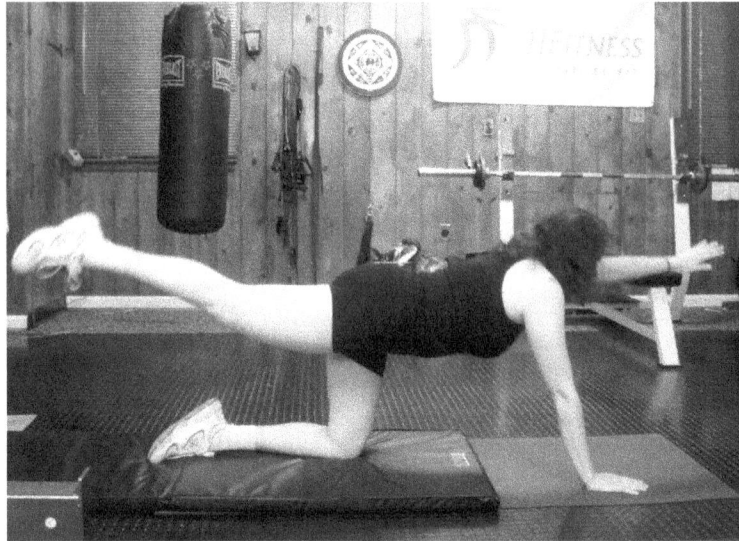

Biceps: **Band Curls**

◊ Stand in good Hara position in the middle of band
◊ Curl to mid chest and return slowly
◊ After 5 reps, hold in isometric position for 5-8 seconds
◊ While you are in isometric position, do a body scan to identify and release all tension, and visualize that your hands are two sides of a perfectly balanced scale. Relax into the exercise
◊ Slowly lower and complete 10 reps

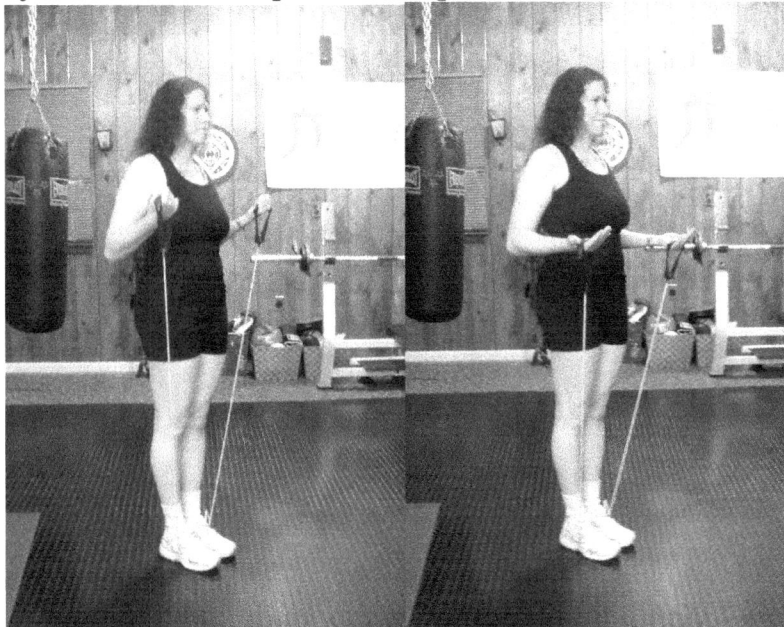

Chest, Triceps, Hara: **Push-Ups on Swiss Ball**

◊ Kneel in front of Swiss Ball
◊ Drape torso over ball and place hands on ground
◊ Walk on hands out till ball is mid thigh
◊ Keep back in neutral position
◊ Keep head in front of hands
◊ Keep hands wide to distribute effort between chest, shoulders and triceps
◊ Slowly bend arms to lower the body, and push up
◊ Visualize that you are a gazelle in the Serengeti dipping your head for a drink from the oasis

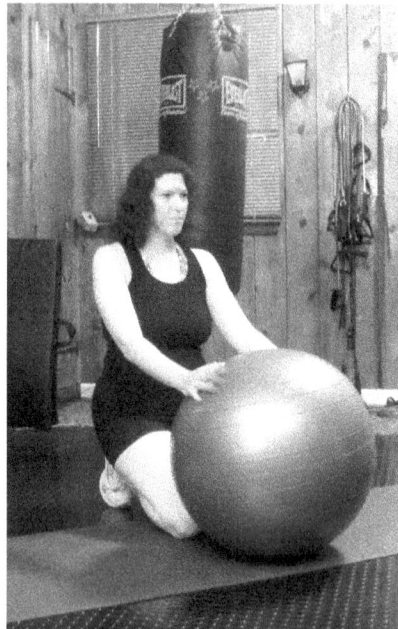

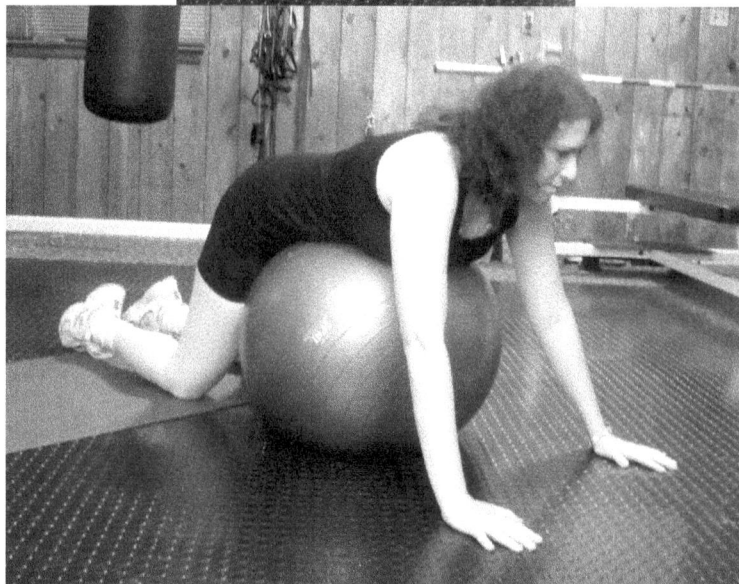

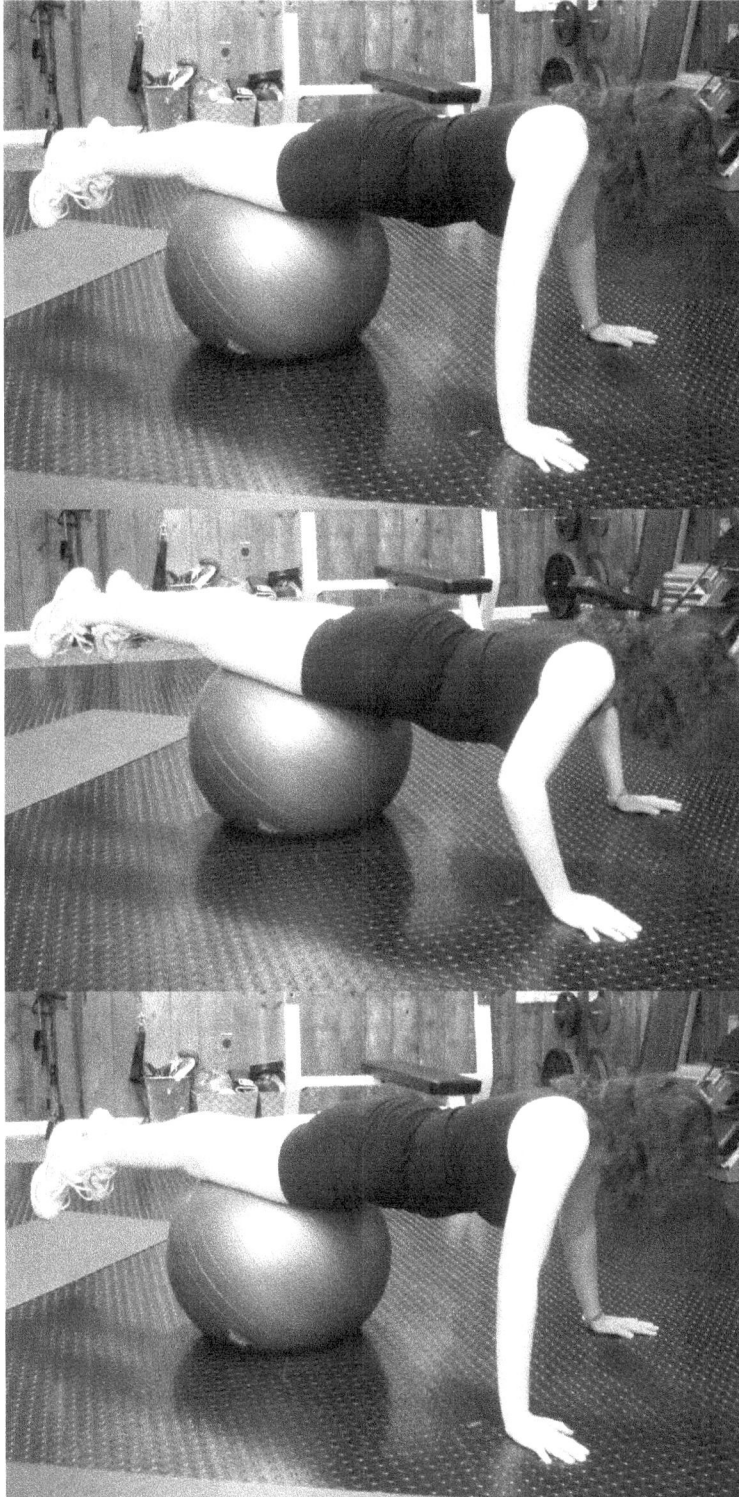

Hara: **Crossovers**

◊ Lay on mat with right hand behind head, left foot crossed over right knee
◊ Place left hand on right oblique
◊ Crunch up and twist, raising right shoulder blade off ground.
◊ Keep left leg still, your elbow wide and chest open
◊ The only goal is to raise the shoulder blade, not to touch the knee
◊ Visualize twisting your torso with every rep
◊ Switch sides

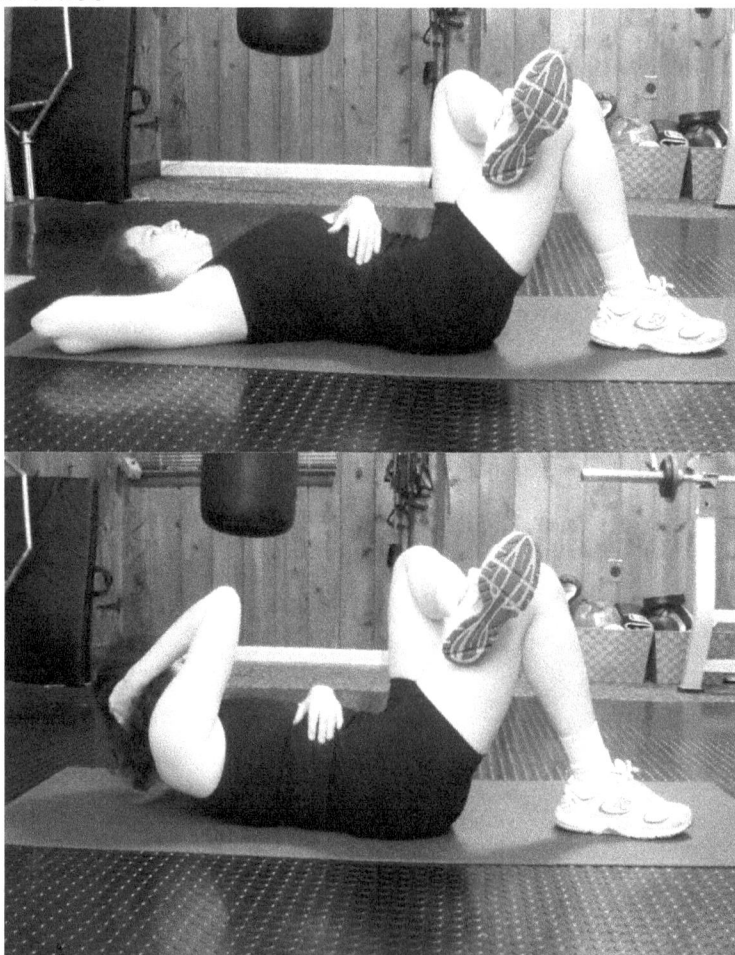

Lats: **Band Low Row**

◊ Sit on floor, legs out flat in front
◊ Keep back straight
◊ Attach band to secure object or have partner hold in the middle of the band
◊ Take band in hands, palms facing
◊ Pull to lower torso, even with belly button. At back position, pause a quarter beat
◊ Visualize two strings attached to your elbows pulling them back
◊ Slowly return

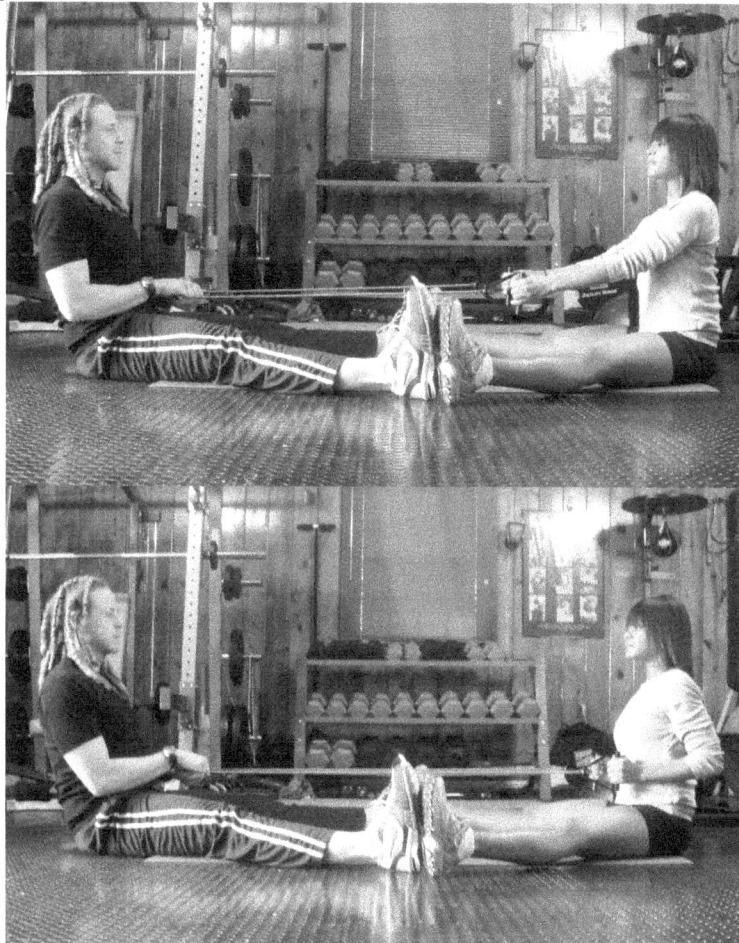

Lats, Hara: **DB Pullover**

◊ Sit on Swiss ball
◊ Take single dumbbell, holding securely between thumb and forefinger of both hands
◊ Establish bridge
◊ Extend dumbbell directly overhead

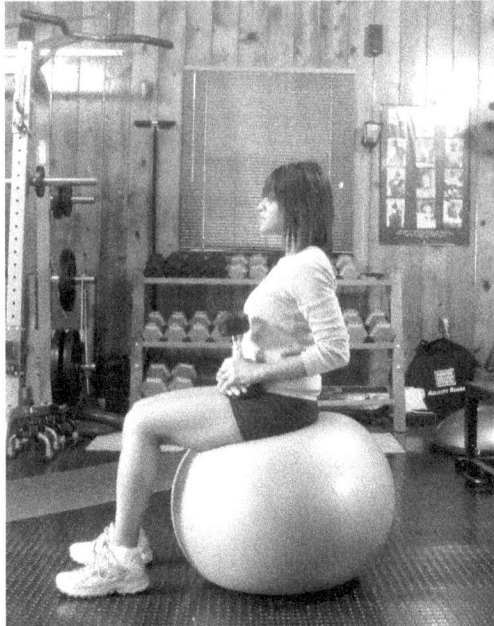

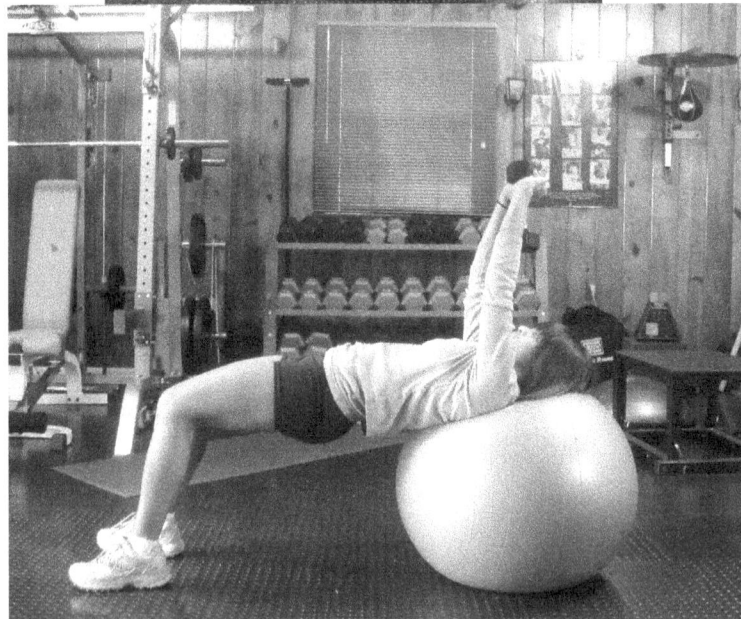

◊ As you inhale deeply, slowly lower dumbbell until a medium stretch is felt
◊ At the bottom of the range of motion, begin breathing out and slowly raise dumbbell in an arc until even with bottom of ribcage
◊ Visualize that the weight is at the end of a long pendulum

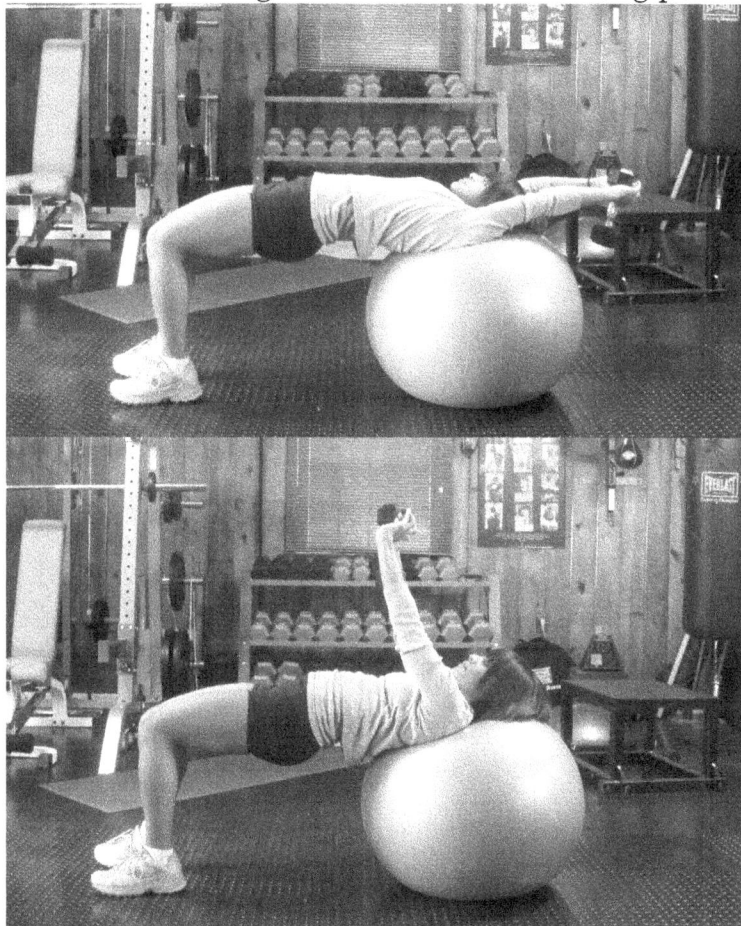

Quads, Glutes: **Step Ups**

◊ Stand in front of step in good Hara position, dumbbells in hands place right foot on step

◊ To step up, move hips back and lean slightly forward. Keep head up and chest open

◊ All effort should be through the foot on the step

◊ Once up, shift weight and use left leg to lower right foot to slowly to ground

◊ Bring left foot down, then reposition on step and repeat

◊ Step pattern is R-R-L-L

◊ Visualize that you are climbing a very steep mountain in extreme altitude with heavy gear on your back

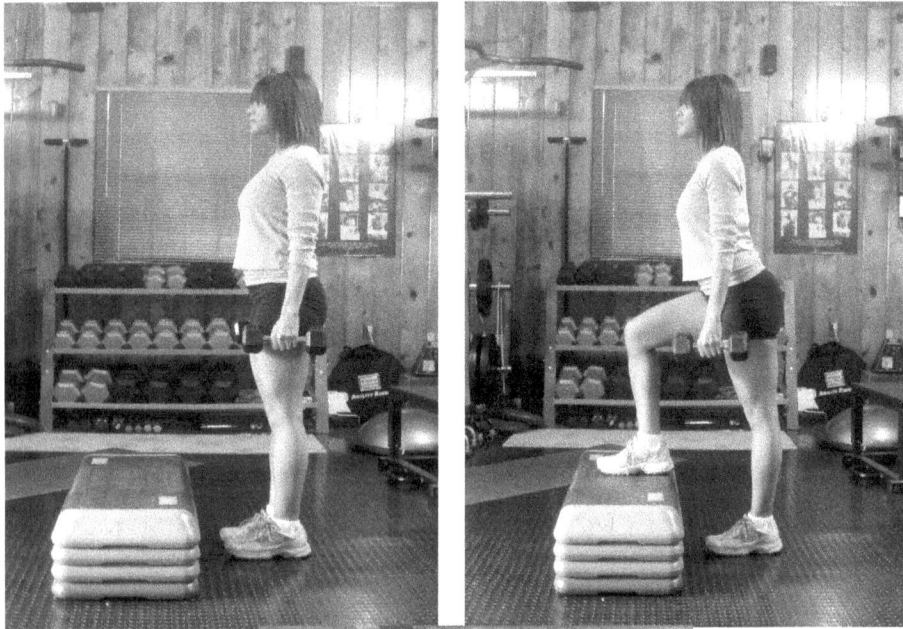

These are not the step-ups of your aerobics class, often done fast to the cadence of music.

GO SLOOOOW!

Step-Ups are one of the toughest exercises ever designed.

HANG IN THERE, you will see results!

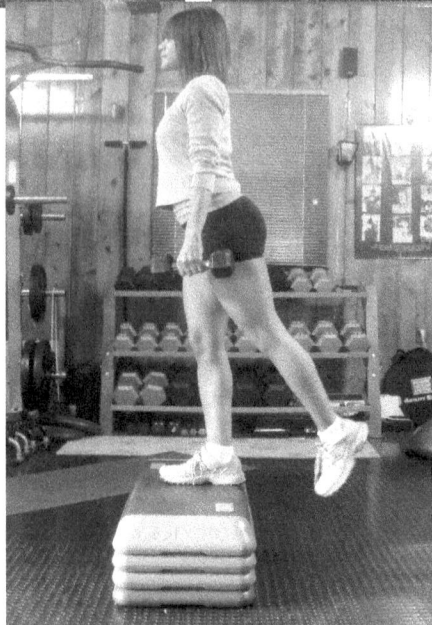

TIP:

If it feels easy, chances are you are "springing up" too quickly by using the leg on the floor, rather than relying on your quad/glutes on the stepping leg.

Focus: **Bridge Track**

◊ Lay on mat and establish a bridge
◊ Extend arms towards ceiling, palms together
◊ Keeping arms straight, slowly move right hand in arc to side

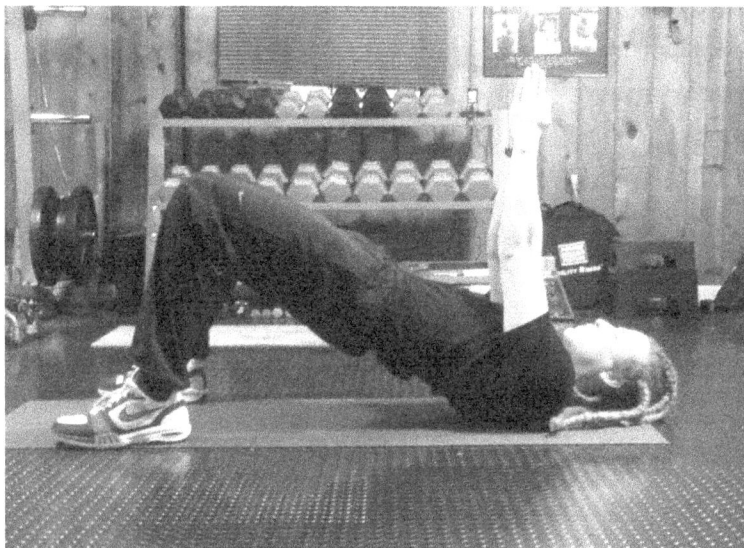

◊ Follow hand with eyesight, turning head
◊ Return slowly and repeat on left
◊ Visualize that your are watching the sun rise and set over the horizon

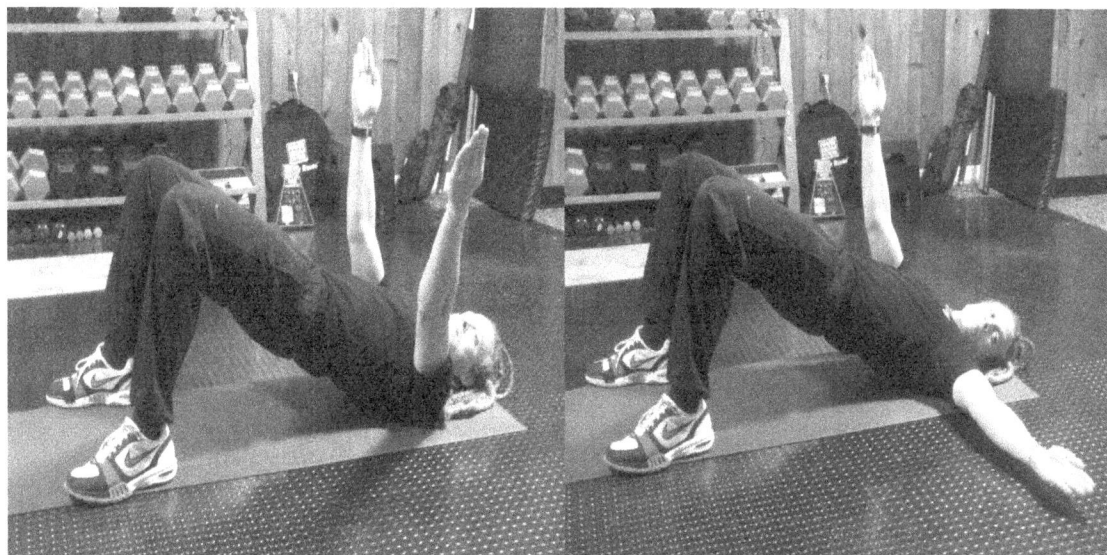

◊ Perform 8 reps (4 reps on each side)
◊ Count to 5 seconds for each rep. Total time for 8 reps should be 40 seconds.

Lats: **Pulldown**

◊ Secure band high over head
◊ Kneel, sitting on heels if comfortable
◊ Take band in both hands
◊ Keep shoulders down and back, head up, back arched
◊ Pull hands to outside of middle chest. Visualize two strings attached to your elbows pulling them toward the floor
◊ Slowly return

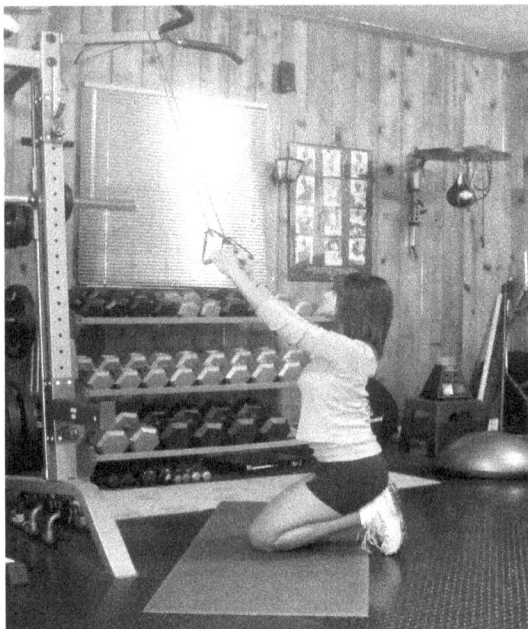

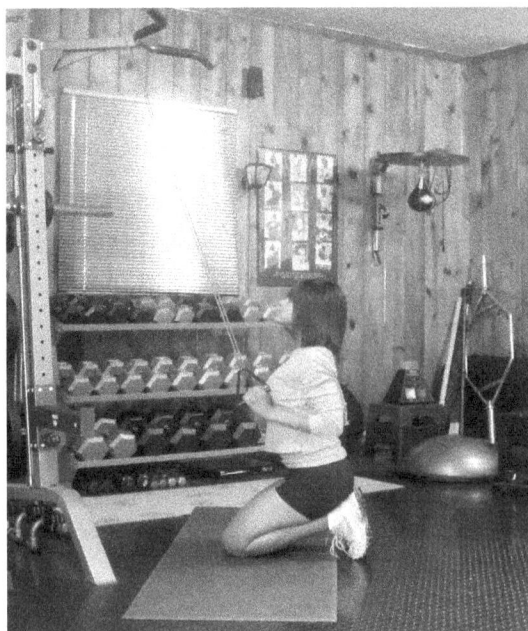

Hips/Hara: **Single Leg Lateral Lift**
◊ Lay on side with hand supporting head

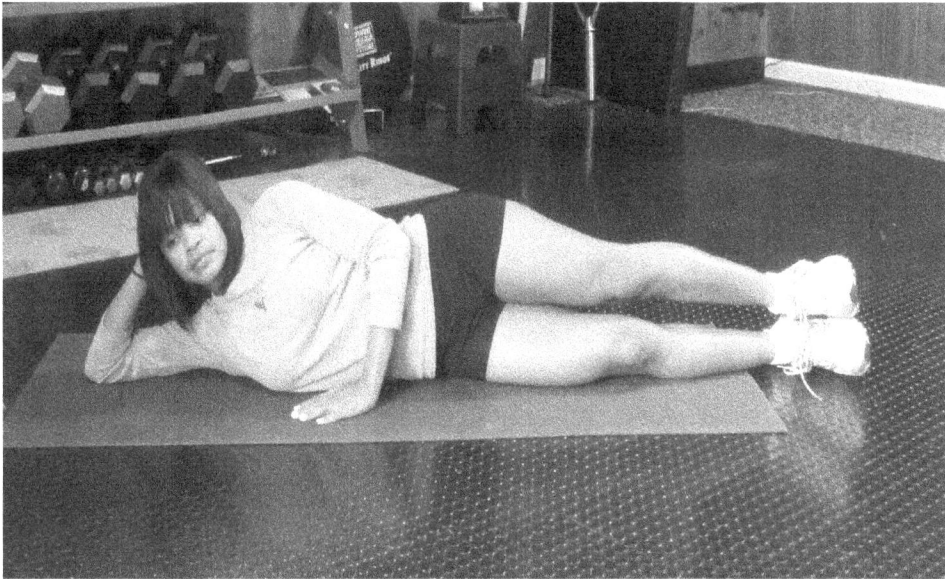

◊ Keeping leg straight, raise to top of range of motion, hold a quarter of a beat, and lower slowly
◊ Maintain body position with hips closed, resist the tendency to rotate forward or back
◊ With every rep, visualize that you are forming a large letter V with your legs

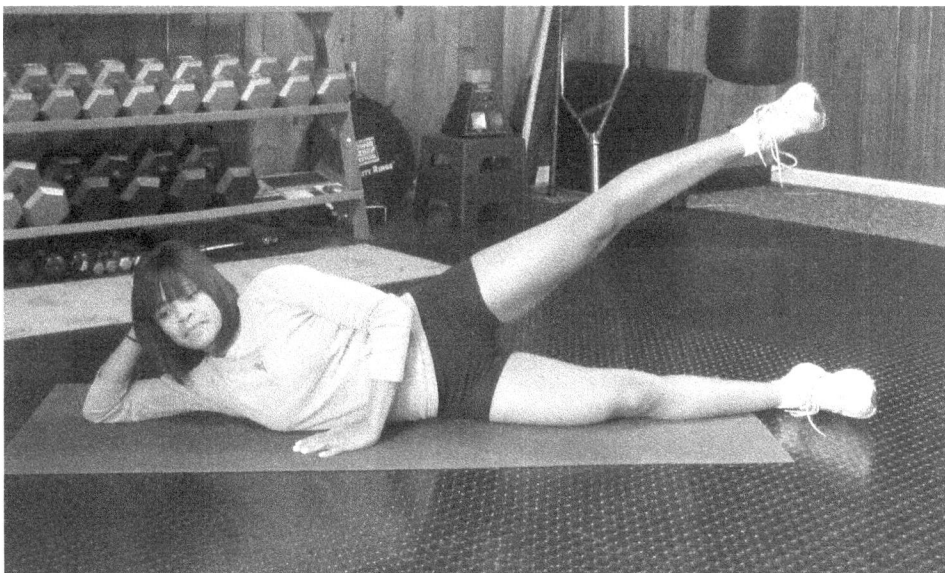

This is another common exercise frequently done to the cadence of music during aerobics class. If you go too fast, you'll lose the benefit of this move. **SLOW DOWN AND LET IT BE HARD. FIND YOUR OWN RHYTHM!**

Hips/Hara: **Single Leg Lateral Lift on Bosu and Swiss Ball**

◊ Kneel beside the balance ball
◊ Drape body sideways over ball, placing bottom hip on ball
◊ Slowly raise and lower top leg, maintaining balance
◊ With every rep, visualize that you are forming a large letter V with your legs

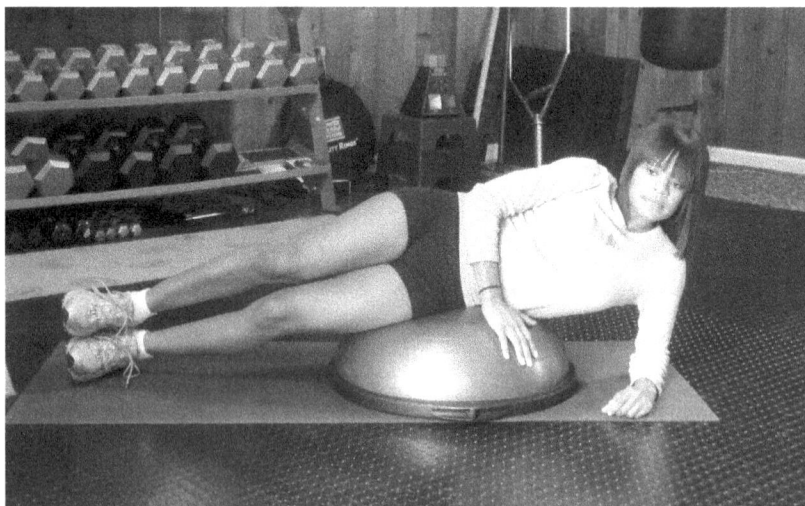

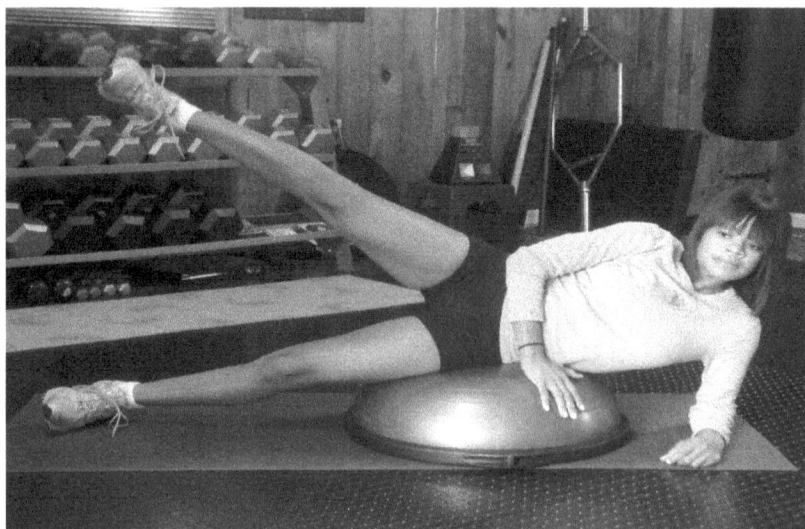

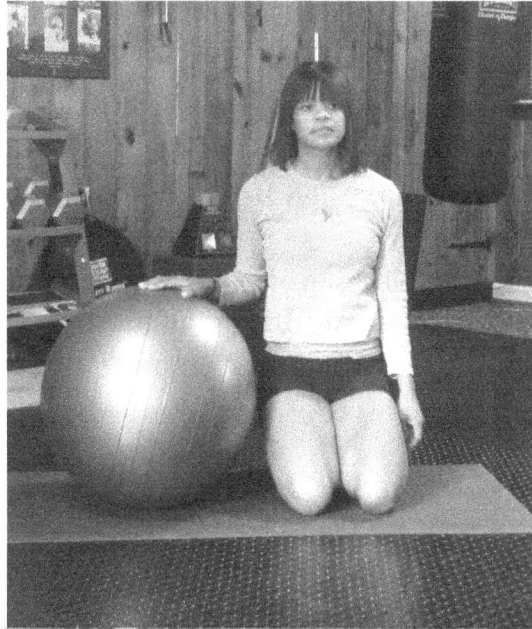

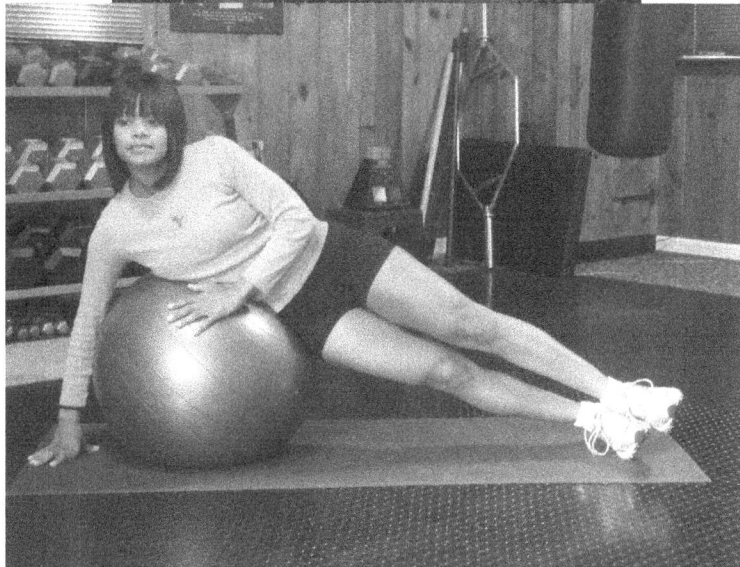

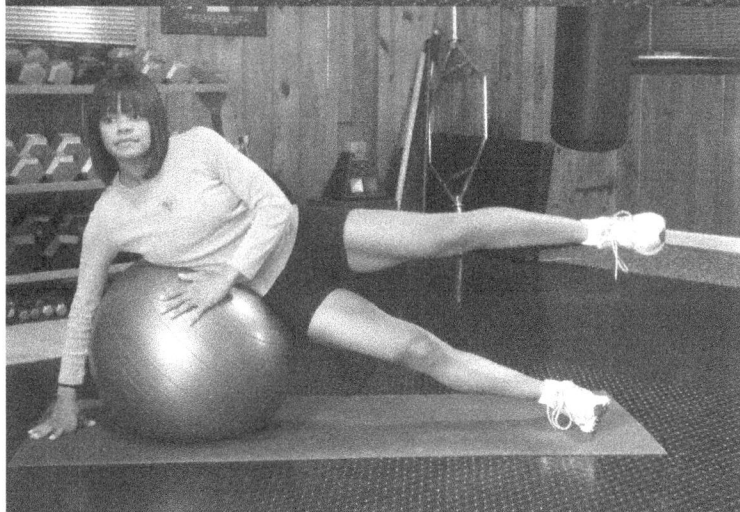

Hara: **Frog Leg Crunch**

◊ Lay on back, soles of feet together
◊ Join hands in front and crunch forward so that your shoulder blades come off the ground. Keep the effort smooth, no jerking!
◊ Breathe a short controlled breath out at top of motion
◊ Slowly return
◊ Mentally focus on the point right below your breastbone
◊ Visualize a gentle wave lifting the shoulders

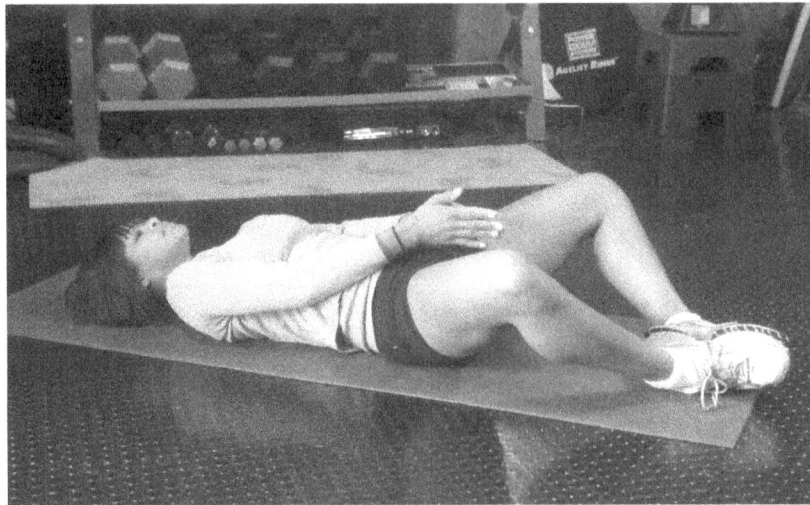

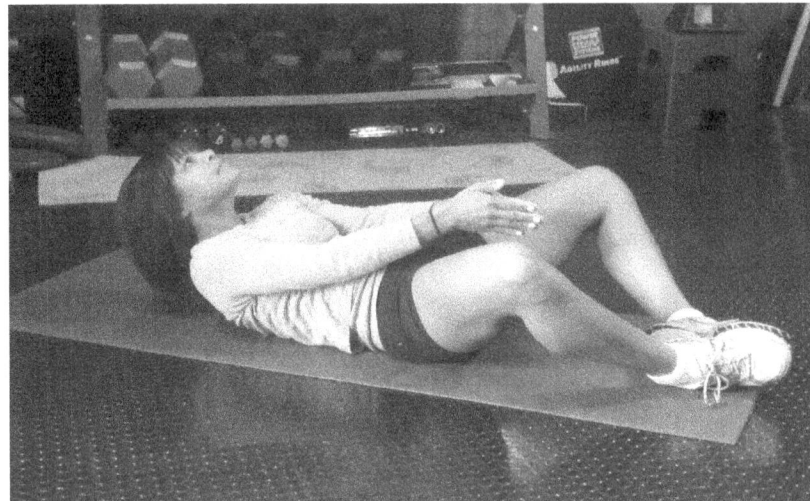

Hara: **Sprinter's Stretch**
◊ Lay on side with feet and knees stacked, arms straight out hands together
◊ Raise top knee as high as possible and rest it on the ground

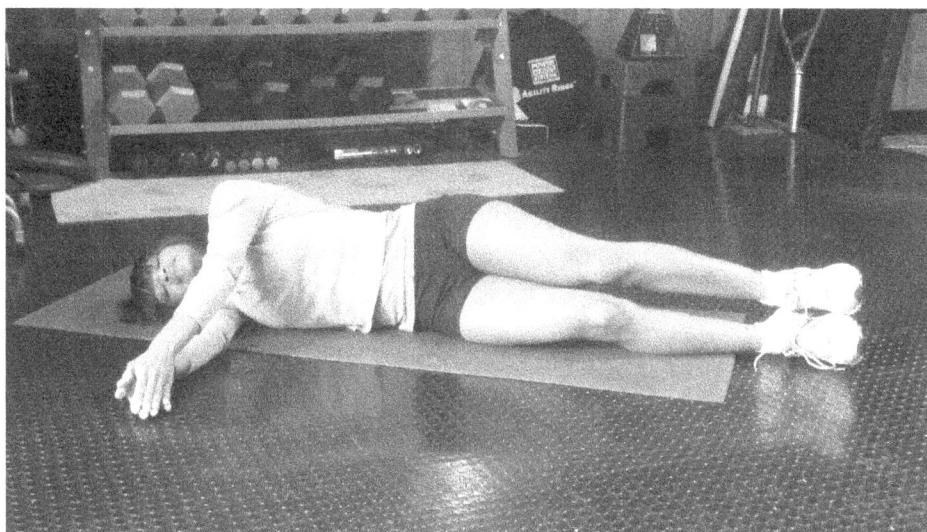

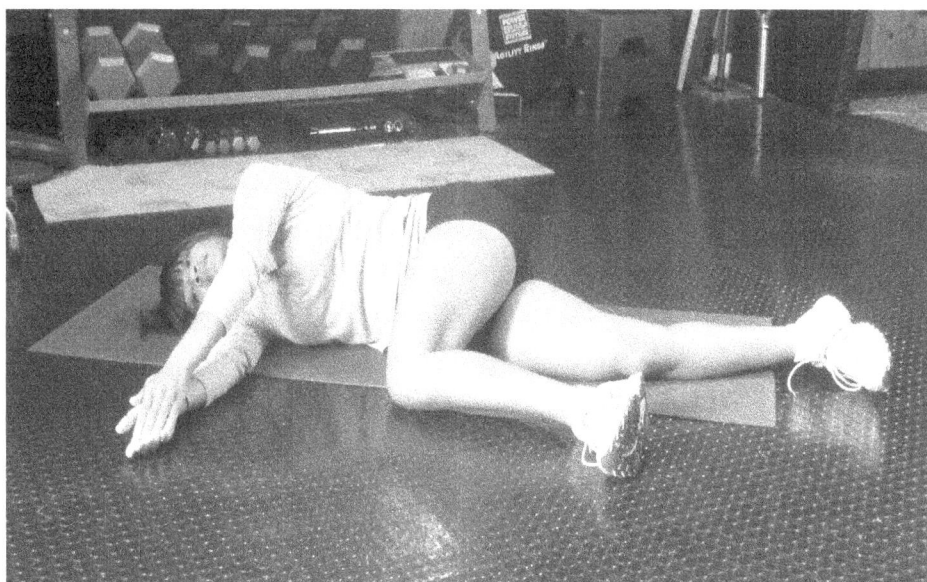

◊ While breathing in deeply, move top hand in an arc all the way over the body to the opposite side. Unless you are extremely flexible, you won't be able to touch this hand to the floor.

◊ You should feel a nice stretch in the chest and lower back. Visualize the muscles of your back becoming Long and Strong. Use this time to appreciate your body and know that you are getting rid of back pain forever!

◊ Hold 20 seconds, breathing slowly, and return

◊ Switch sides

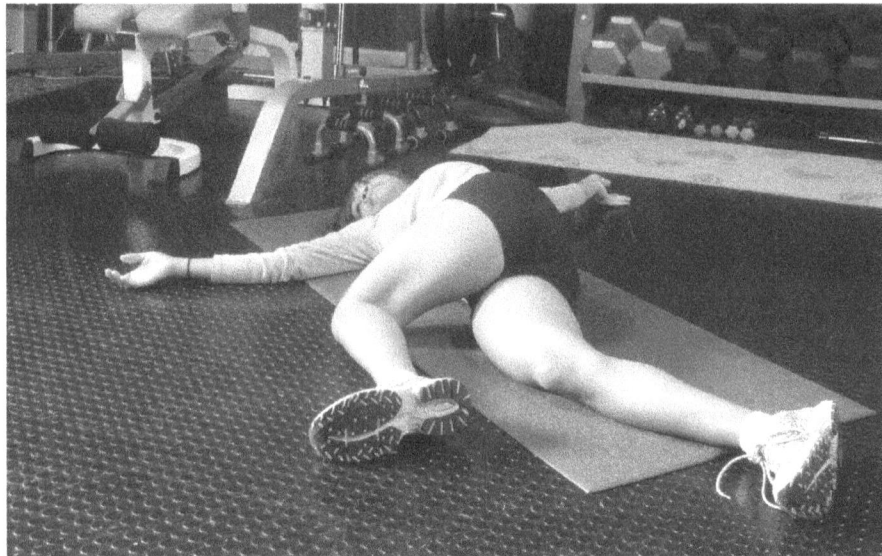

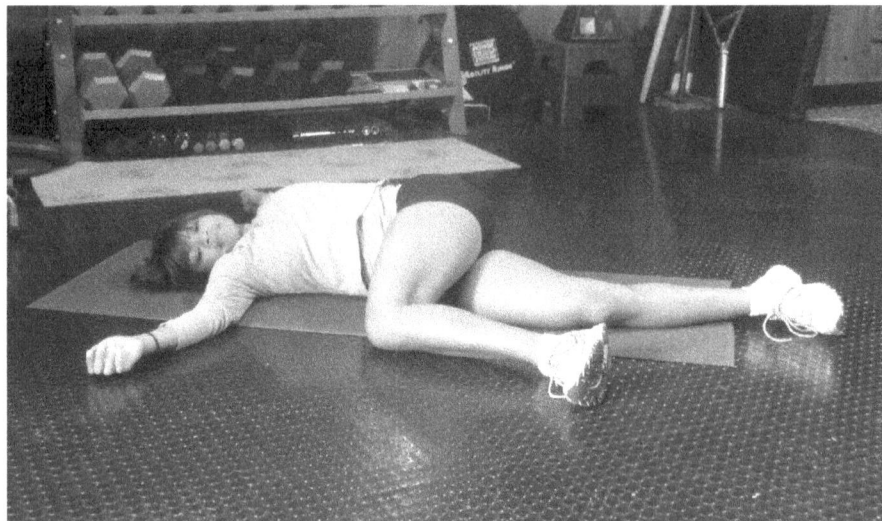

Breathe into your stretch!

Focus: **Tip Toe Tracking**

◊ Stand on tip toes
◊ Extend arms straight out, hands together
◊ Staying on toes, slowly move right hand to side, following hand with eyesight
◊ Turn head to follow hand
◊ As you open your hand, visualize that your are opening your body and spirit to positive change. Establish a space within which you can feel and visualize perfect balance and movement!
◊ Return slowly and switch

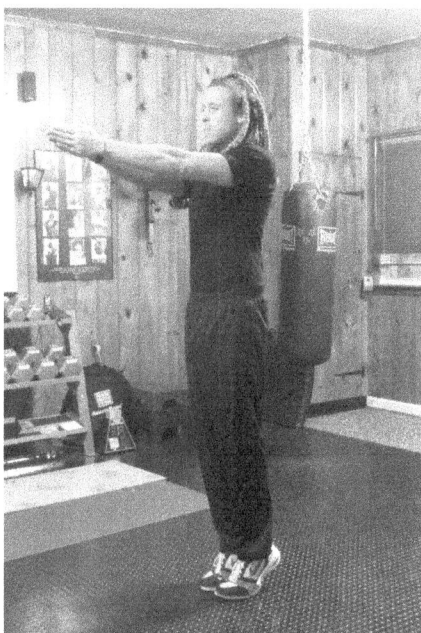

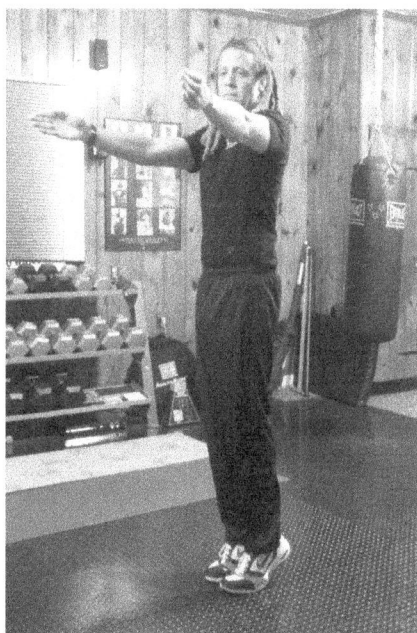

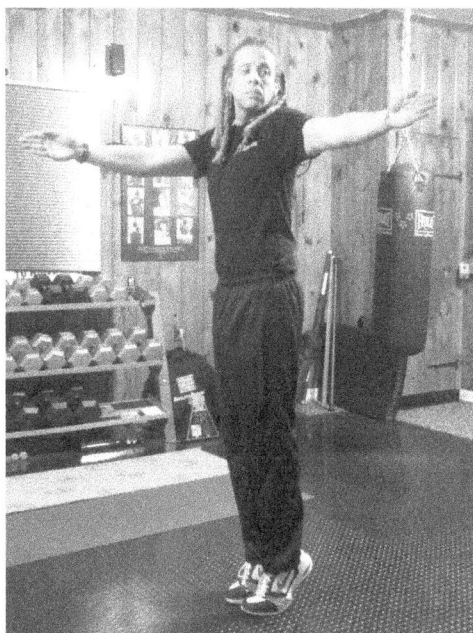

Glutes, Quads, Hara: **Donkey Kick**

◊ Come to all fours position on mat
◊ Place band around one foot and take in both hands
◊ Extend banded foot straight back, feeling tension on the band
◊ Visualize that you are giving a mighty kick in slow motion
◊ Slowly return and repeat

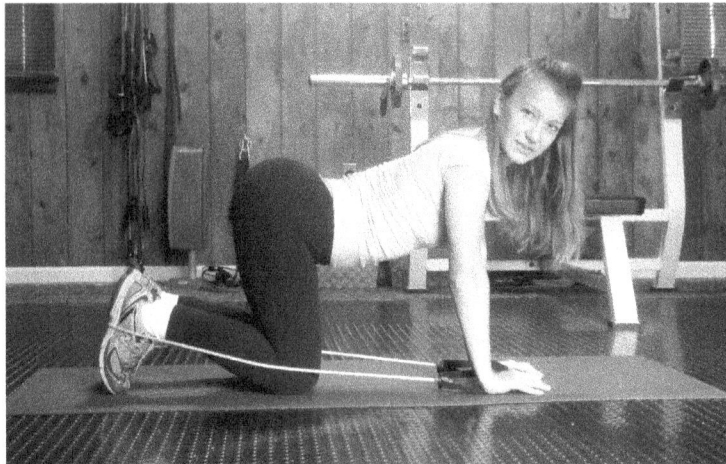

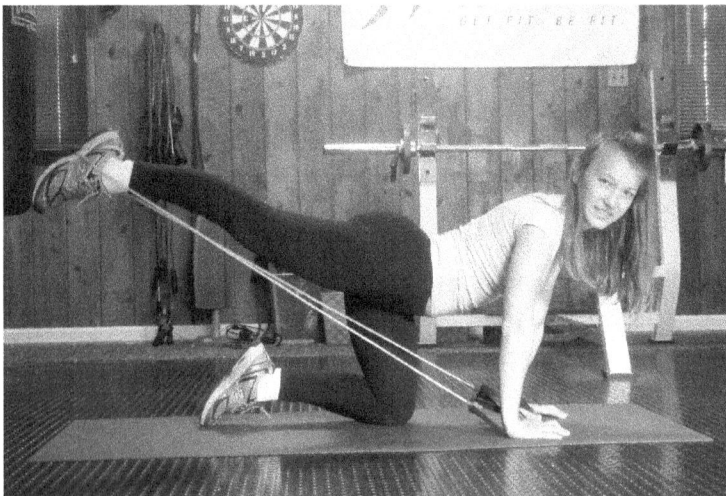

TIP:

Keep your kicking foot flexed so that it holds onto the band securely and you avoid a painful SNAP!

Triceps, Chest: **Dips**
◊ Sit on bench or chair
◊ Extend legs to straightened position
◊ Place hands on each side of your butt on bench

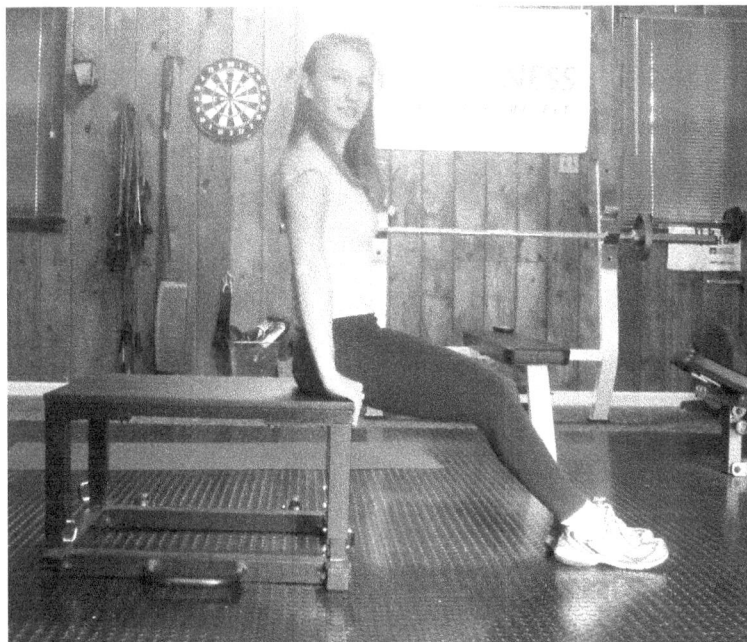

◊ Keeping arms straight, slowly slide off bench

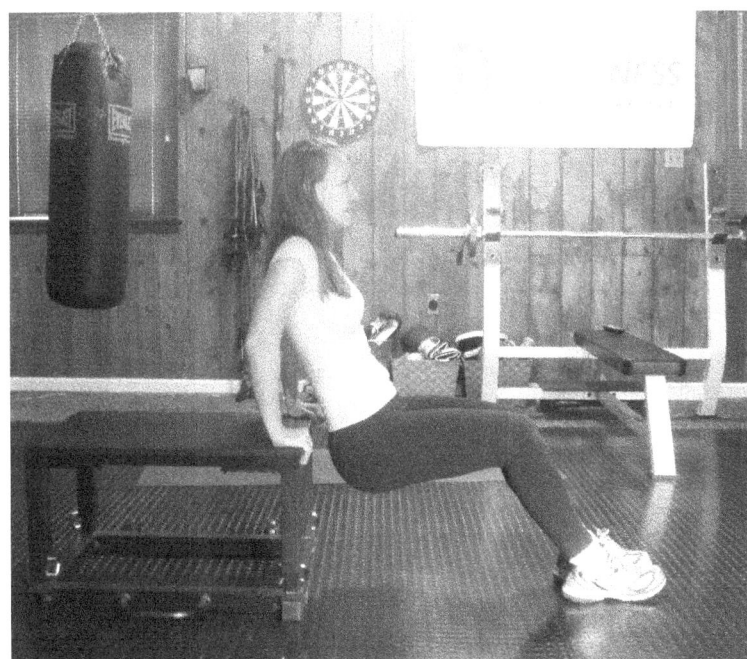

◊ Slowly lower body towards the floor.
◊ Do not go too far too quickly. Visualize that you are lowering yourself into a swimming pool of very COLD water and get a feel for how low you can go.
◊ Push back up until arms are straight. Repeat exercise.

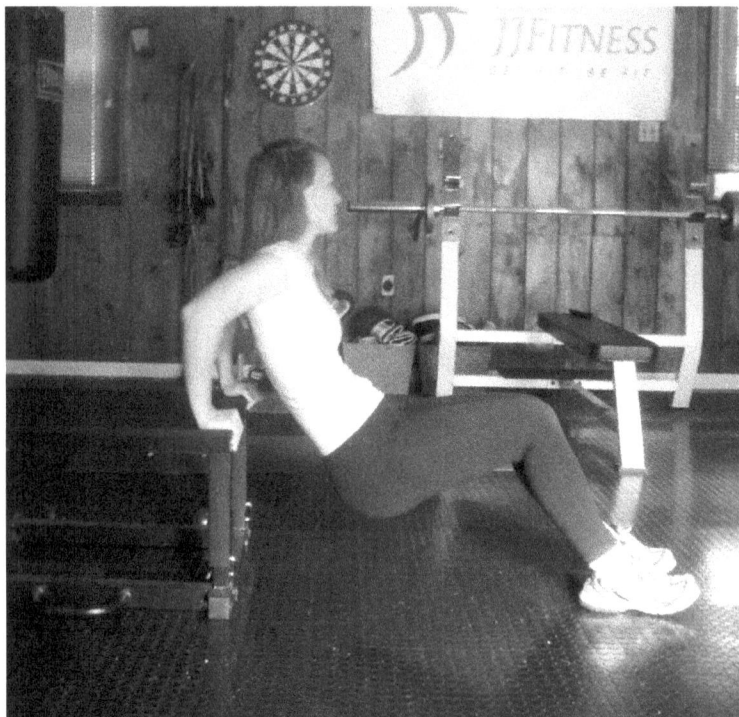

Depending on what parts of your body where you hold your weight, dips can be very challenging especially when first getting started.

TIP:

Try doing partials (not going too low) or perhaps fewer reps
until you feel comfortable,
but always try to challenge yourself!

Hamstrings, Butkus, Erectors: **Romanian Dumbbell Pull**

Preparing to pull:
- ◊ To learn the movement stand in good Hara position
- ◊ Place hands on thighs and arch back
- ◊ Bend at the waist, moving hips back and slide hands down thighs
- ◊ Keep head up and shoulder blades together
- ◊ Visualize that there is a wall behind you that you must touch with your butt, but keep your back arched
- ◊ When good stretch is felt in hamstrings, press through heels to slowly return

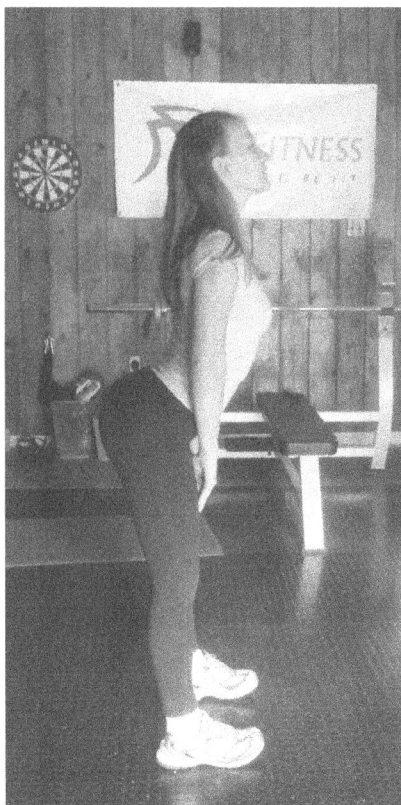

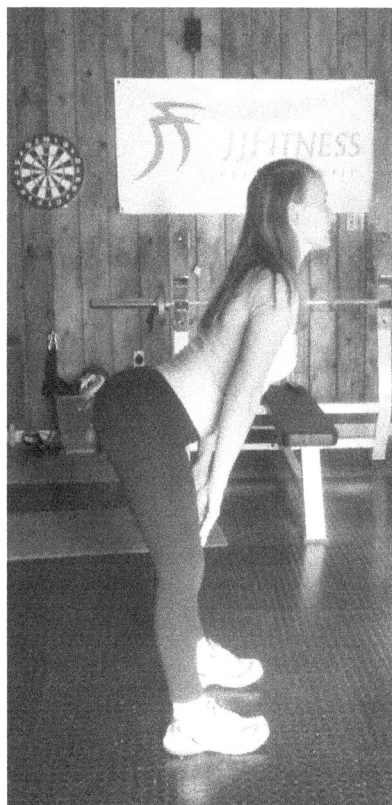

Now that you have practiced the form for the dumbbell pull, you can try adding some light weight.

The Romanian Dumbbell Pull is an all time favorite exercise in the JJ's Way Training Program! It's both physically and mentally challenging, because of the need to focus on GOOD FORM throughout the entire body.

◊ Stand in good Hara position with dumbbells in hand
◊ Place hands on thighs and arch back
◊ Bend at the waist, moving hips back and with hands holding dumbbells (still sliding down the thighs), reach for the floor very slowly.
◊ Keep head up and should blades together
◊ Visualize that there is a wall behind you that you must touch with your butt
◊ When good stretch is felt in hamstrings, press through heels to slowly return

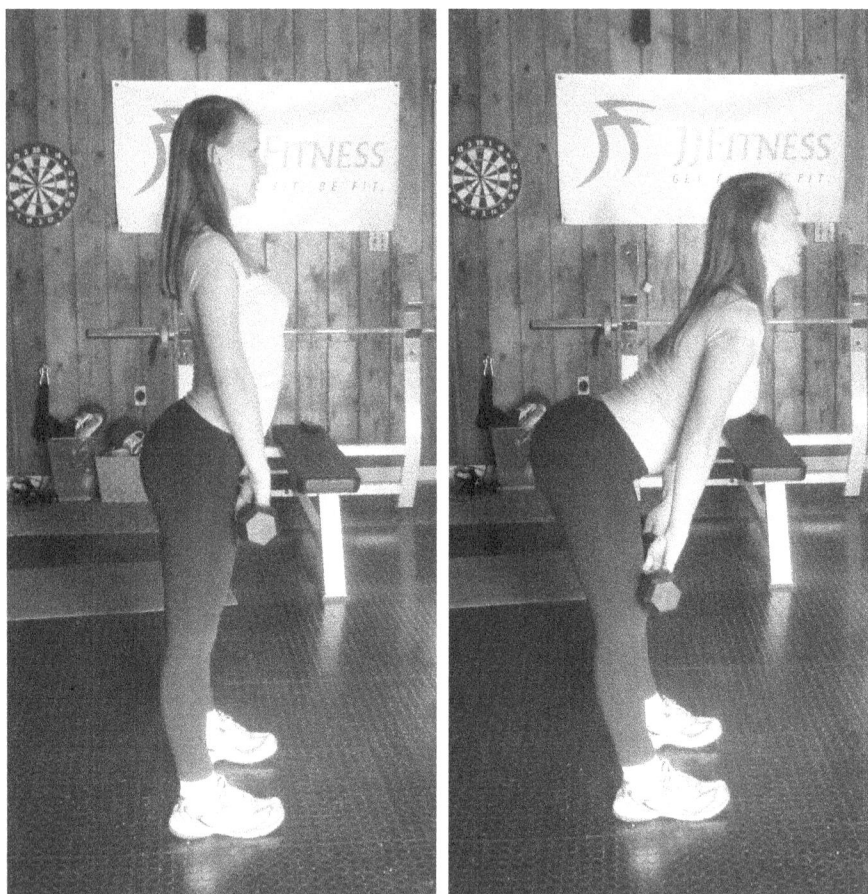

TIP:
Try testing your form by standing 8-10 inches from an actual wall. When you do the exercise, try touching your butt to the wall as you go down!

Hara/Focus: **4 point balance on Swiss Ball**

◊ Lean in front of Swiss Ball with both hands and knees leaning on ball.

◊ Slowly push forward with both hands and come to balance position on ball. Find your center of gravity. You may need to press down more with your right or left hand (or both), or shift weight back towards your hips.

◊ Squeeze your legs together to hold onto your position on the ball.

◊ Hold for 30 seconds

◊ Come off of ball in balanced position

◊ Visualize that you are a highly trained acrobat performing at an amusement park. Use this time to think good things about yourself

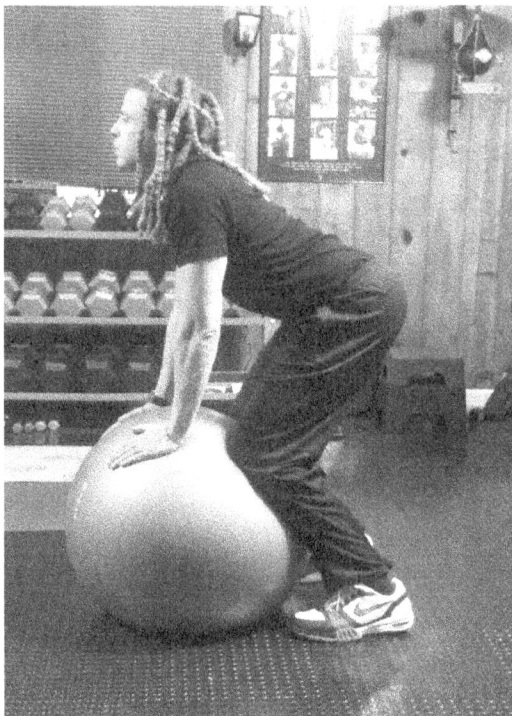

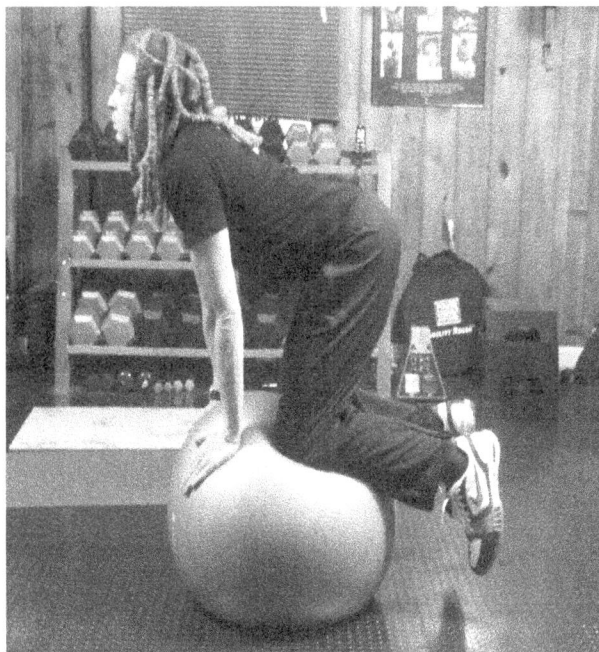

◊ Stay relaxed!

**Balance improves with practice,
keep core pulled in, stay breathing,
pick a spot in front of you and FOCUS**

**If you don't get it the first time,
the second time will be much better!**

Chest: **Dumbbell Flye**

◊ Sit down on Swiss Ball and get into a bridge position with dumbbells
◊ Extend dumbbells directly overhead, palms facing

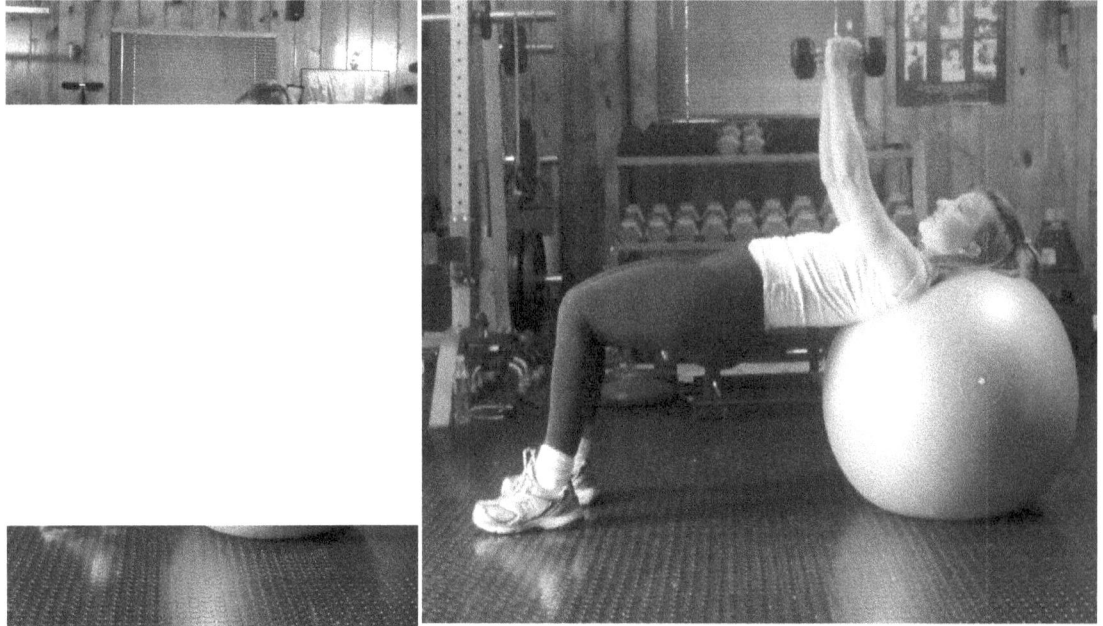

◊ Keeping a 5 degree angle in arms, slowly lower while breathing in until a slight stretch is felt in chest. Visualize hugging a big bag of rice.
◊ Don't go too low, and keep your arms LONG and STRONG.
◊ When you get to the bottom position your hands should be in line with the mid to lower chest.
◊ Return arms slowly to overhead position, breathing out

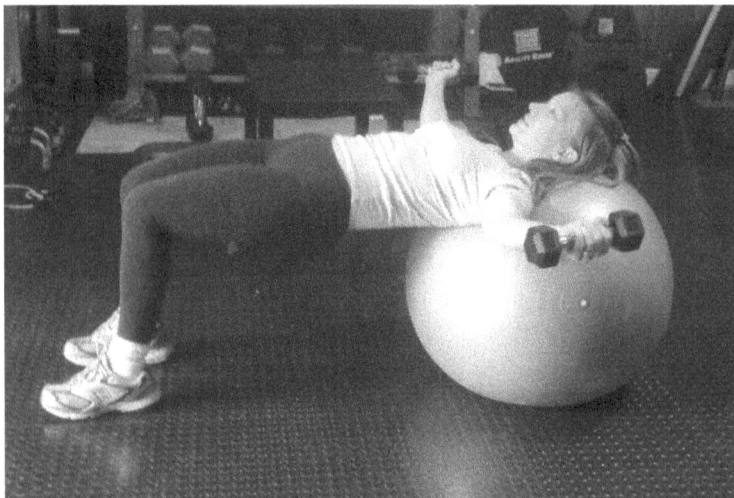

Adductors: **Band Leg Adduction (or "Sweep the Stoop")**

◊ Attach one end of band to a secure object close to the ground
◊ Attach other end around the forefoot.
◊ Move away from attachment so that there is tension on band
◊ Balance with opposite hand, raise foot and move laterally across body, keeping your foot straight
◊ Visualize that you are literally sweeping some leaves off a stoop with your foot.
◊ Slowly return and repeat

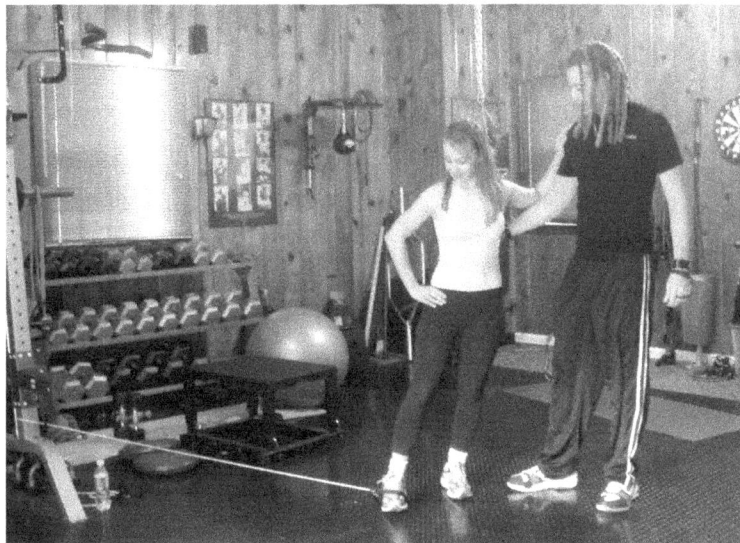

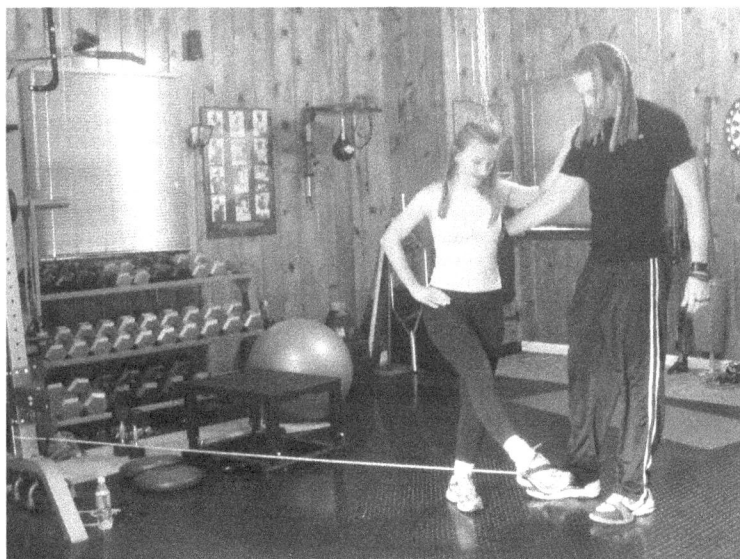

Hara: **Plank**

◊ Kneel with elbows and knees on mat

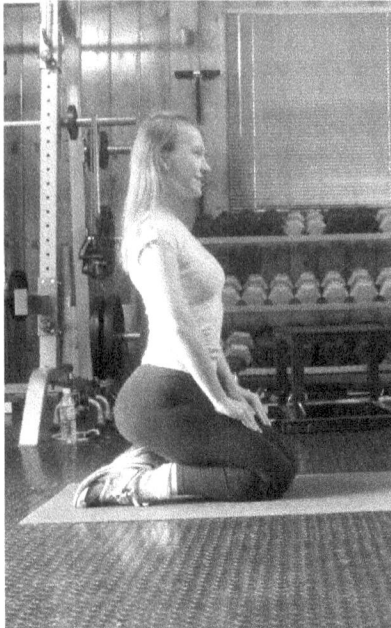

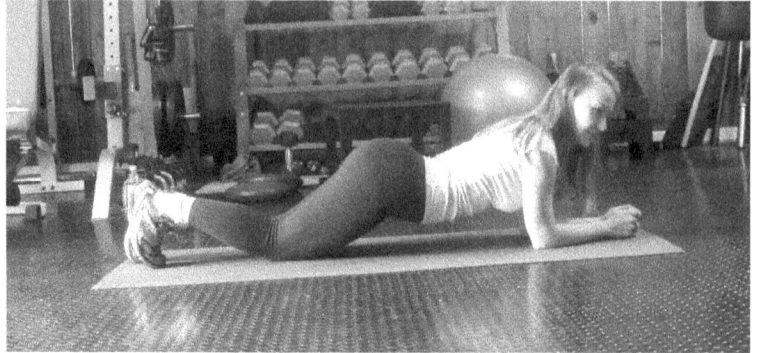

◊ Come to "plank position" on toes and elbows (body is stiff as a board)
◊ Stay breathing and relax
◊ Hold for 20 seconds
◊ Visualize that your body is a strong beam of wood, capable of providing support for a whole house. Use this time to focus on your goals
◊ Slowly lower

Your body may shake or quiver during the Plank exercise.

Don't worry, you will adopt!

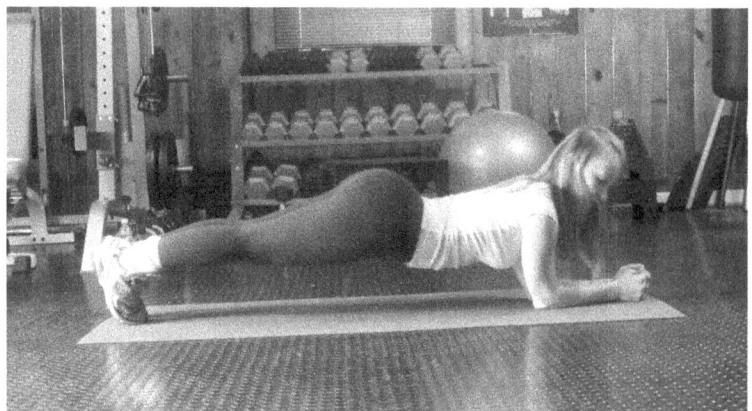

Focus: **Tree Pose**
◊ Stand with sole of foot on inside of opposite knee
◊ Find a stationary spot in front of you to focus on
◊ Relax and breathe
◊ Hold for 20 seconds, switch sides
◊ For added challenge, raise arms above head and join hands

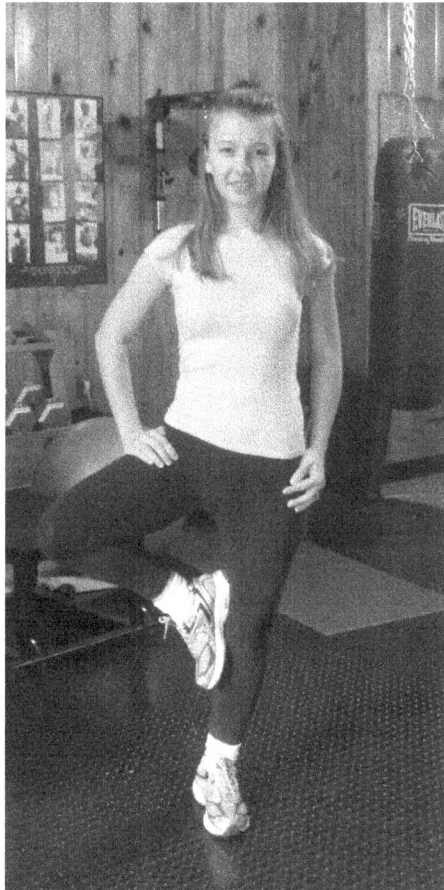

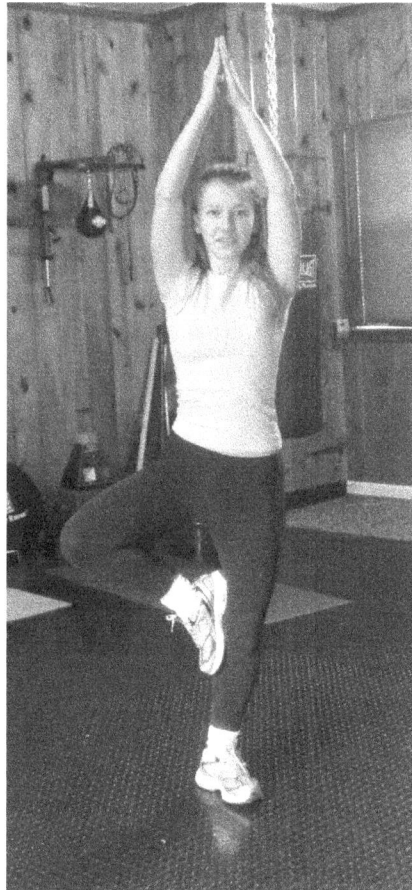

Visualize that you are a tall tree in a quiet woods. Your foot is rooted to the ground and you are in perfect balance. There is a slight breeze, but your solid trunk allows your arms and legs to adjust while your position remains undisturbed.

You are growing every minute of every day and realizing your full potential!

Chapter 11: The Perfect 6

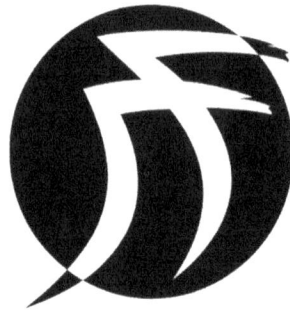

So: How have you been eating?

I used to ask this question of my clients at the beginning of every session. What was their answer? "Pretty Good." "Not Bad" or if they were naughty "Not so good" None of these answers tell us anything of value!

The answer to this most important question should never be 'good' or 'bad' but quantitative.

In JJ's Way we use a scale of 1-6 to rate how we've been eating.

A 6 on the scale is perfect, never missing. 5-6 meals a day, every 3 hours, with the right amount of protein, Low Glycemic (LG) carbs, and vegetables.

A 1 on the scale is 2 meals, usually a lunch and dinner, big meals, followed by a healthy dose of sugar, or a pizza binge etc.

> *"GET TODAY RIGHT!"*

If a trainee eats at a 4-6, is training within proper heart rate zones, and weight training 2-3 times a week, WEIGHT LOSS and FITNESS IS GUARANTEED!

JJ's Way Perfect 6 Scale –

How does the Perfect 6 Scale Work?
Each day, give yourself a rating on a scale from 1-6. "6" - Ate every 3 hours with proper food perfect portions "5" - Ate 5 meals including breakfast, not perfect portions "4" - Ate breakfast, 3-4 meals, some starchy carbs but no sugar "3" - Ate breakfast and 2 more meals, starchy carbs each meal "2" - Skipped breakfast, ate 3 times, no attention to what I ate "1" - Ate twice, something greasy and something sweet, skipped breakfast

Copy this chart into your Discovery Journal

Today's Date	6	5	4	3	2	1

Look for patterns in your eating! Note the patterns and Discover ways to be consistent in the 5 and 6 range.

Chapter 12: Weeks 5-8 Training

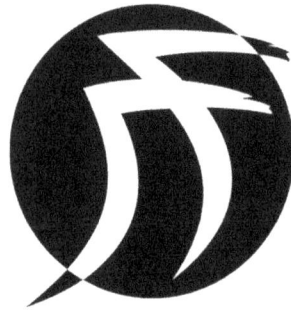

Congrats, you've made it a month! Chances are you've already seen and felt change – you have more energy during the day, are sleeping better at night, the pants you wear most often are just a little looser in the waistline.

And The Best is Yet To Come!

Most likely you've missed a workout or two. No worries. It's always about what's next that matters. You can step on the scale regularly - 1-2 times per week, but not daily - to see how well you're doing. Whether the change in numbers is a big or a small one, keep working the JJ's Way program.

Note that the exercises on Day 3 are NOT done in supersets.

JJ's Way 3 Qualities of Training are:
Consistency: the regular habit of exercise

> *Trust the Process*
> *Trust Your Trainer!*

Focus: optimism, concentration and mindfulness during exercise

Patience: It's a Process. Enjoy the Process!

JJ's Way 3 Rules of Nutrition are:
NO REFINED SUGAR

No 'FAST' or 'JUNK' food

No alcohol

Let's Keep Training!

Indicates "Super Set"
Indicates "Hara" exercise

DAY ONE

PAGE	ACTIVITY	REPS	SETS	BREAK
67	Warm up	5 min	Zone 1	
81	Toe Touches	8	2	no break
83	DB Lateral Raise	12		
84	DB Military Press	12	3	60 - 20 sec
89	Front Hold	30 sec		
87	Hip Raise	30 sec	2	30 sec
94	DB Chest Press	12	3	60 - 20 sec
96	Band Flye	12		
106	Push ups	8 to 12		
91	Modified Leg Raise	12 - 15	3	10 sec
79	Cardio	20 min	Intervals	
67	Cool down	5 min	Zone 1	
69	Stretch	5 min		

DAY TWO
Rest and Diet

DAY THREE

PAGE	ACTIVITY	REPS	SETS	BREAK
67	Warm up	5 min	Zone 1	
92	Side Bends	10 sec	3	no break
101	Band Squat	12	3	60 - 20 sec
85	Band Stationary Lunge	12	3	60 - 20 sec
90	Calf Raise	15	3	60 - 20 sec
103	Quad Extension with arm	25 - 60 sec	2	30 - 10 sec
112	Step Ups	24	2	60 - 20 sec
115	Single Leg Lateral Lift	10 - 15	2	60 - 20 sec
108	Crossovers	12 - 15	3	5 sec
	NO CARDIO!!!			
67	Cool down	5 min	Zone 1	
69	Stretch	8 min		

DAY FOUR

PAGE	ACTIVITY	REPS	SETS	BREAK
67	Warm up	5 min	Zone 1	
81	Toe Touches	8	2	no break
114	Pulldown	12		
109	Low Row	12	3	60 - 20 sec
110	Pullover	12		
113	Bridge Track	8	2	15 Sec
105	Band Curls	5 hold 10		
137	DB Hammer Curl	10	2	60 - 20 sec
138	Tricep Extension	12		
118	Frog Leg Crunch	12 - 15	3	5 sec
119	Sprinter stretch	20 sec	2	no break
79	Cardio	25 min	Zone 2	
67	Cool down	5 min	Zone 1	
69	Stretch	5 min		

DAY FIVE
Rest and Diet

DAY SIX

PAGE	ACTIVITY	REPS	SETS	BREAK
67	Warm up	5 min	Zone 1	
121	Tip Toe Track	10	2	20 sec
122	Donkey Kick	12		
139	1 Arm DB Military Press	12	3	60 - 20 sec
125	Romanian DB Pull	12		
127	4 point balance	1 min	2	15 sec
140	1 Arm DB Chest Press	12		
141	Jump Rope	30-60 sec	2	60 - 20 sec
123	Dips	12		
130	Plank	20 - 60 sec	2	10 sec
131	Tree Pose	2 min	1	
79	Cardio	25 min	Zone 2	
67	Cool down	5 min	Zone 1	
69	Stretch	5 min		

DAY SEVEN
Rest and Diet

Weeks 5-8 Exercises

Biceps: **DB Hammer Curl**

◊ Sit on Swiss ball with dumbbells
◊ Sink down to semi squat
◊ Relax arms to bottom position, elbows against ball, palms facing in
◊ Curl to top position
◊ Top position should be less than 180 degree angle to floor
◊ Visualize your arms as pistons in a car engine
◊ Lower slowly

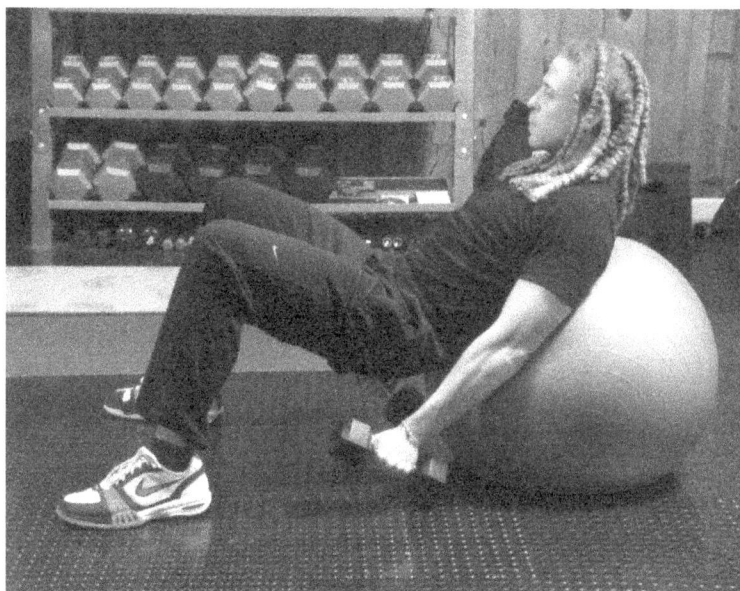

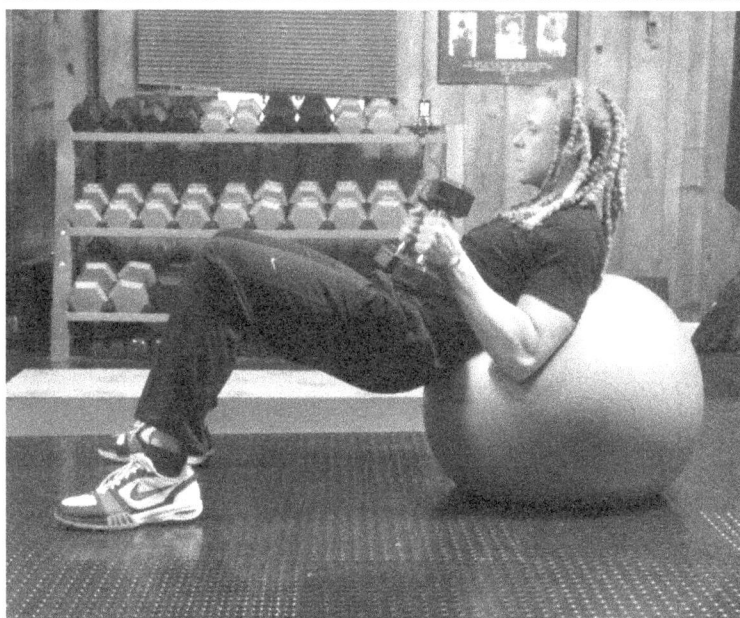

Triceps: **Triceps Extension**

◊ Stand with one foot on band, step through with other foot
◊ Bring hand up to behind the head and join band
◊ Establish position with upper arm perpendicular to floor

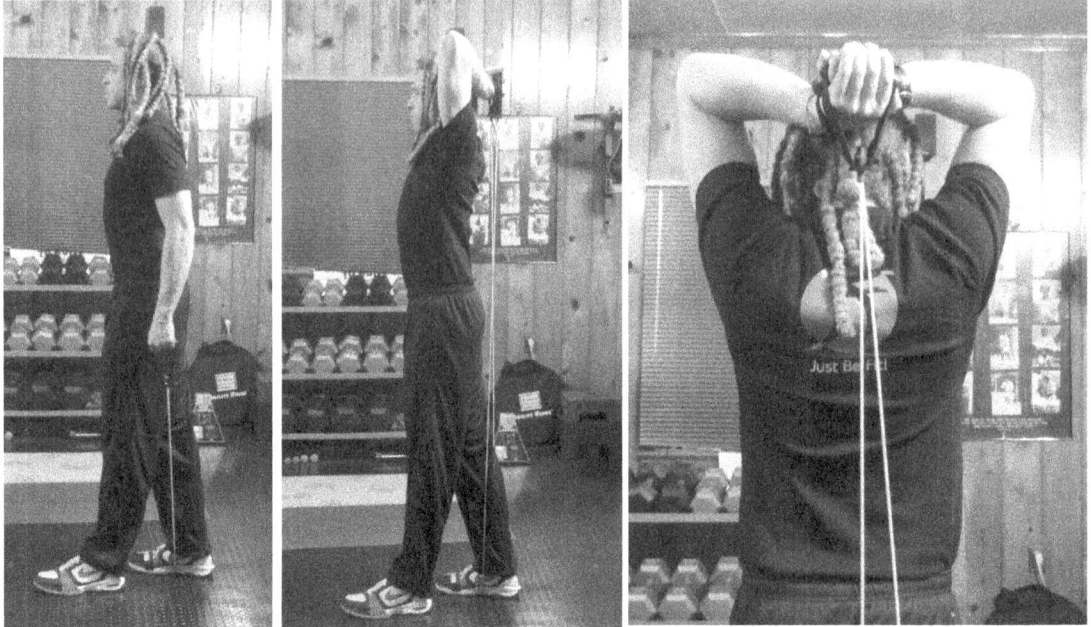

◊ Keeping your Hara tight, straighten arms to ceiling. Visualize bringing water up from a deep well
◊ Lower slowly

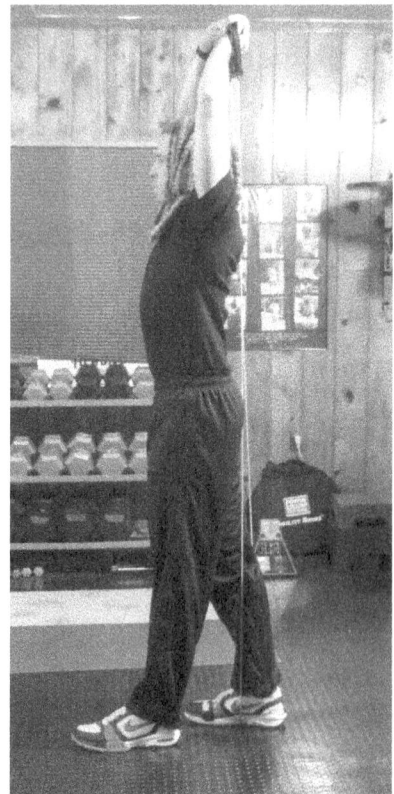

Chest, Hara: **1 Arm Military Press**

◊ Sit on Swiss ball with one dumbbell
◊ Bring dumbbell to start position
◊ Keeping torso upright, press dumbbell to top position
◊ Visualize raising a slow motion punch to the ceiling
◊ Lower slowly

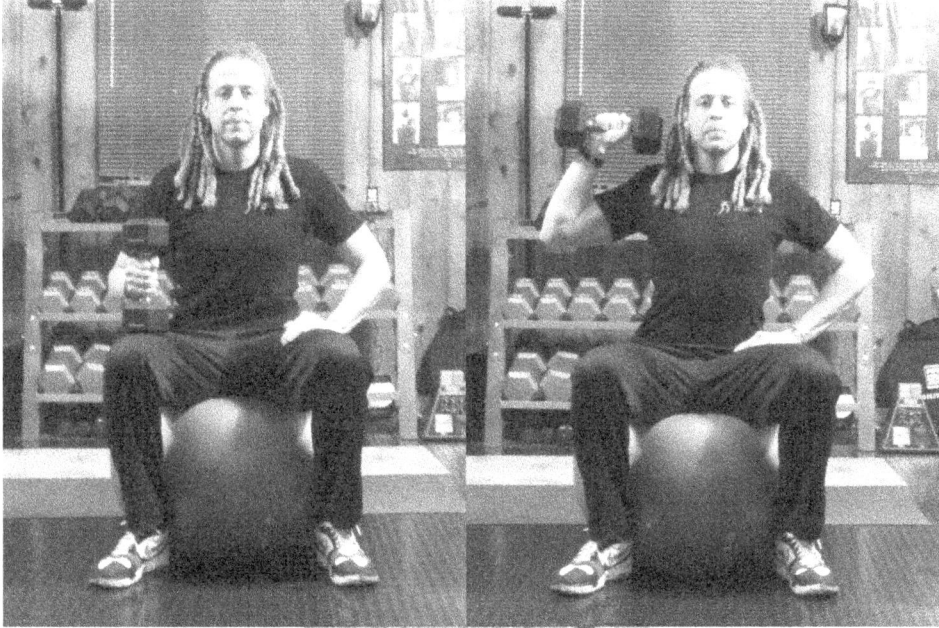

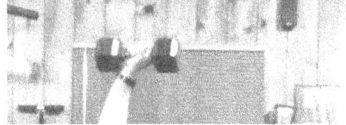

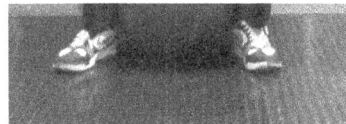

Chest, Hara: **1 Arm Chest Press**

◊ Sit on Swiss ball with one dumbbell
◊ Establish bridge position
◊ Bring dumbbell to start position
◊ Keeping Hara position, press dumbbell to top position
◊ Visualize a slow motion punch to the ceiling
◊ Lower slowly
◊ At end of set, use Hara to sit up

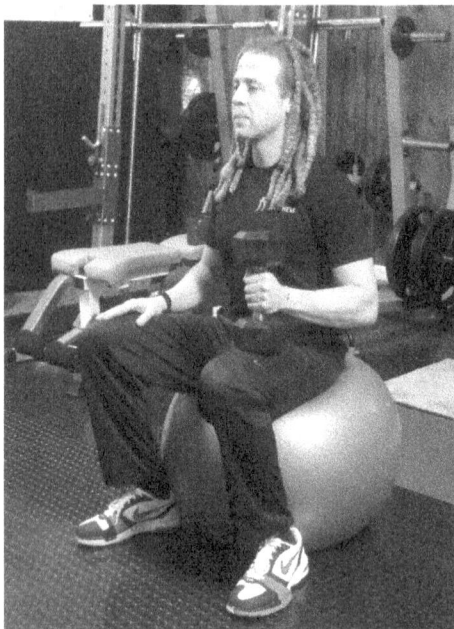

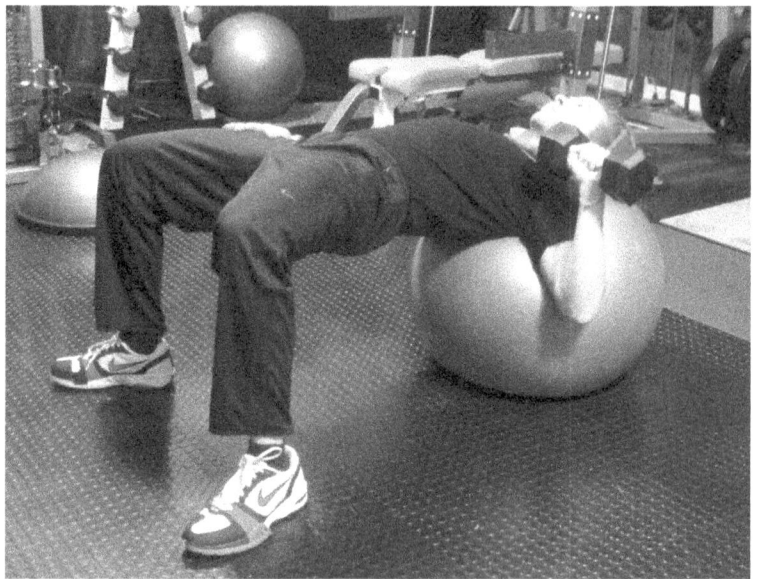

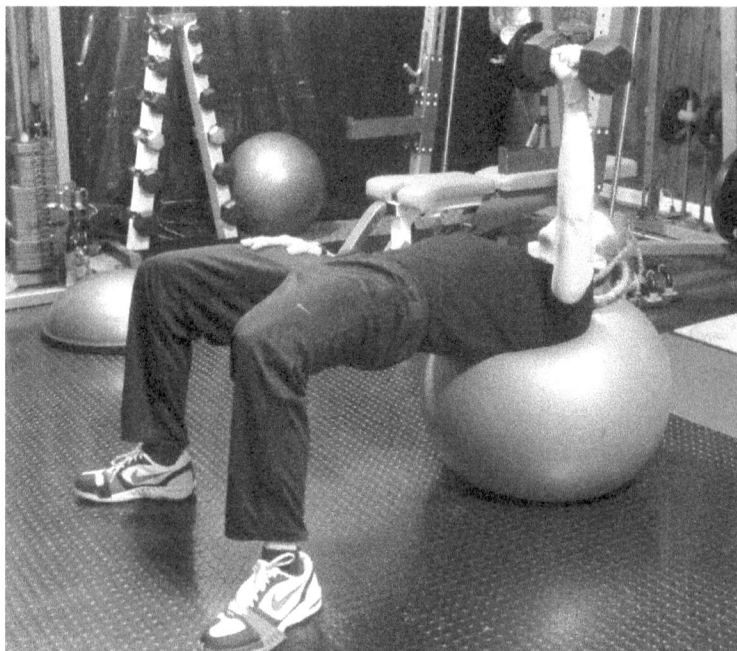

Full Body: **Jump Rope**

Jump roping is the best full-body workout that exists!

A single low jump per rope swing. With rope jumping LESS IS MORE. Ideally the jumps should be ½ to ¾ inch off the ground. The control required to jump less than an inch while landing softly on the balls of the feet is a *whole body movement*.

The Two Basic Techniques:

1. Bounce Step
   Both feet together

2. Alternate Foot Step
   Alternate feet like jogging in place
   Keep feet in front

It takes discipline and practice to master rope jumping. The body AND mind must gradually adapt.

The first goal is 30 seconds with consecutive jumps for the two basic techniques.

Begin with 5 to 10 jumps per set for a total of 5 sets. Jump for 1 minute, resting as needed.

Gradually increase the reps for each set by 10 to 25 per set.

Even missteps and catches of the rope develop the kinesthetic and proprioceptive senses, enhancing agility, balance and coordination.

See the Discovery of JJ's Way DVD for further instruction and demonstration

Chapter 13: Lifestyle, Nutrition and Weight Loss

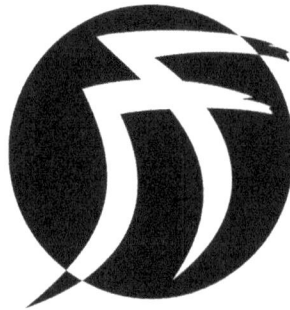

JJ's Way 10 Ten Point Plan for Fitness and Wellness

1. Build your meals around protein, healthy fat, and vegetables
2. Eliminate Sugars and Starches (refined grains). .
3. Consume more omega-3 and much less omega-6 oils. Avoid trans-fat.
4. Avoid Alcohol but if it is a must, do red wine in 4-6oz quantities.
5. Eliminate processed foods. Cutting SS alone is not enough. You have to cut the junk!

In most cases, no matter what they say on the package, the food industry is not your friend.

6. Drink plenty of water
7. Sleep is a weight loss drug. Get plenty of Sleep
8. Exercise at the appropriate intensity and duration 3-5 times a week. Training is the best way to boost a metabolism.
9. Do stress release, joyful things. Pleasure is a nutrient!
10. Being healthy well and fit is a process. Enjoy the Process!

A Nutrition Repetition

To repeat, when insulin levels rise: → the less fat you burn,
→ the more sugar you store in fat cells, along with the extra fat that the liver makes from sugar.

When insulin is present, your body fat cannot be "burned" or "released" to any significant degree , therefore...

The more sugar you store, the fatter you get!

To compound the problem, the more fat you gain, the more insulin resistant you become – it becomes harder and harder for you to process the sugar you take in.

But your pancreas still puts a lot of insulin in your blood.

When you have consistently high levels of insulin, and the glucagon can't keep up, the body will bring in some helper hormones, cortisol and adrenaline, to help. This leads to a pre-diabetic condition.

Why your "helper hormones" are really LIFESTYLE Hormones

CORTISOL is a catabolic (reducing) hormone, secreted by the adrenal gland. Its primary function is to keep your blood pressure from getting too low.

Cortisol also helps Glucagon counter to effect of insulin.

Most importantly, cortisol is connected to Lifestyle. Feelings of stress, anxiety and depression trigger its release.

ADRENALINE is also a catabolic hormone secreted by the adrenal gland. Its primary function is to keep your heart beating.

Cortisol and Adrenaline are known as the stress hormones. Both are primitive hormones – the fight or flight response – that serve to as a "turbo" system for emergency response.

For most of our modern lifestyles, the stress hormones are in our systems far more than is necessary. ***Rather than fending off a Saber Tooth Tiger, dealing with daily stresses*** like traffic, problems at work, financial issues, arguments with family members and friends. triggers your adrenals to work overtime.

Although they are essential to life function and are helpers to Glucagon, too much of the stress hormones is a bad thing. They weaken the immune system and break down muscle.

When muscle is broken down, **your metabolism slooooooows to a crawl** and you reduce the number of muscle cells that will accept sugar, leading to that sugar being stored as fat.

Finally, the body sends in a hormone to protect itself from too much muscle breakdown: INSULIN!!!

<u>Your goal</u> is to keep excess levels of the adrenal hormones out of your bloodstream, because too much cortisol and adrenaline triggers insulin.

It is important to remember than too much cardio activity causes the release of a lot of cortisol and adrenaline. This is why the JJ's Way program keeps cardio to a manageable level.

ALSO, the stress hormones send powerful messages to the brain to "refuel", leading to stress eating.

AND stressed out people are usually insulin resistant.

STRESS MAKES YOU FAT!

TURNING THE SHIP AROUND...

You can turn the ship around TODAY. The BIG 3: Type II Diabetes, High Blood Pressure, and likelihood of heart disease are all **reversible** and **preventable**!

Insulin resistance is also reversible.

You are not in the minority. 75 percent of our population has some degree of insulin resistance.

As soon as you start losing weight JJ's Way, you stack the hormonal deck in your favor!

SWITCHING FUELS

The purpose of eating JJ's Way is to switch your body from a sugar burning to a FAT BURNING MACHINE!

Soon your body will burn fat for fuel almost exclusively, you will have increased energy and a noticeable sense of well-being. You'll feel great!

JJ's Way of nutrition is one of life's charmed gifts! Following it will truly feel like a breath of fresh air!

The end result of your conversion to JJ's way will be a dramatic shift your body's the insulin/glucagon ratio, indicating an overall shift from a glucose (sugar) based metabolism to a fat-based metabolism. JJ's Way *is* the metabolic advantage.

Remember, fat cells are stubborn, active cells that attempt to protect their own existence unless there is overwhelming action to the contrary, at which they will submit and go along with the program.

As soon as you stick with JJ's Way for 7-14 days, your cells start to become insulin *sensitive* (the opposite of insulin resistant), improving as time elapses. Before you know it, you will have become one of those people who **uses** food for energy and not storage! All the protein you eat increases your metabolic rate and the heat of your body is turned up! And if Sugars and Starches are sufficiently limited, the majority of the fuel the body needs for its day to day operations will come from fat!

Now you have flipped the metabolic script. Now you are a FAT BURNER!

One Size Fits All – *Not!*

The truth is that there is no single diet is for everyone.

Just like there is no perfect dress for all body types, there is no perfect one-size-fits-all diet. Everyone is fundamentally different on metabolic, genetic, and chemical level, and each body responds differently to different types of food.

The fancy term for this is Biochemical Individuality. So the next time someone asks you why aren't you on the South Beach or Atkins or Weight Watchers Diets, raise your eyebrows wisely and say "because I'm biochemically individualistic!"

No two people respond the same way to anything – not to life, not to medicine, not to food, not to diet.

Also remember, your body is different every day. Lifestyle and hormonal cycles account for this.

Good News: everyone benefits from adding protein to every meal, eating smaller meals more frequently, and changing their Sugar and Starch carbohydrates to "real carbs."

> *Practice mindful eating – don't do other things while you're eating, taste and experience your food.*
>
> *Invest in the time to do it!*

JJ's Way and cutting your SS's is a strategy, not a religion. Sometimes life situations - such as the holidays or a family vacation - demand a slight detour. The point is that the JJ's Way strategy doesn't change, even though your tactics might from day to day or month to month.

Strategy is more important than will power in JJ's Way.

It is important to remember that you are trying to make changes on a continuum. It does get easier, but there will be bumps in the road.

The name of the game is the right direction, not perfection.

Weight loss is about taking control of your life.

Weight management is a medium by which you can practice mastery of your mind, your body, your environment.

Master weight management and master your life.

It's never over till you say it is!

The only limits are those you believe in.

Enjoy the process!

Chapter 14: Bumps in the Road

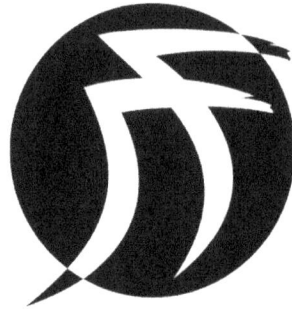

"There is no stasis. Every day you are living a little bit more or dying a little bit – which one will you do today?"

80 percent of trainees will stop training within 3 months. So if you make it through the program in this book, then you are in the top 20 percent.

But there will be bumps in the road: times when you feel like eating poorly and not working out.

Here are a few things to consider:

EVERYONE has Self Doubt. The discovery is how to overcome. Use the fear that is within you.

Recognize and honor the vanity you posses.

Desire and Fear and Vanity are the greatest 'real' motivators.

EVERYONE experiences "Failure". This process is about redefining Failure, recovering, and moving on. At a higher level of resistance training we know that "the moment of failure is the moment of value." The same goes for life!

NONE OF US has enough time. The discovery is employing a little time management to get your meals prepared and your workouts done. Recognize the difference between a reason and an excuse.

Sometimes you will feel good and sometimes you will feel bad, or have an ache, or an imbalance. There are literally about a million factors that figure into your current state of being!

Just Remember: The body is a mystery.

And: The body will remain a mystery.

If you feel lethargic and it is time to train, you should ALWAYS warm up fully before deciding whether or not to train.

There is a difference between standard soreness/tightness, which one can train through, often well, and deep muscle soreness, which indicates the muscle is still in repair and should definitely NOT be trained.

During a setback you need to be mindful that losing weight is an emotional process.

Take a minute to answer this question:

*What else will I be losing
with my weight loss?*

Answers could include:

◊   My current set of close friends with whom I overeat.
◊   My favorite sweatshirt
◊   My protection from unwanted attention

Beware The Soother

Almost everyone is aware of the effects from a trauma which is easily defined: a terrible accident, a death, war, natural disaster, divorce, losing your job. But few of us are conscious that trauma is interwoven into each of our lives from the beginning.

While living our lives we inevitably experience pain as a result of experience: a rejection, invalidation, anger/rage, sexual trauma, failure. There are many origins of trauma.

To minimize the pain from trauma we often do whatever lessens it the quickest.

This quick-fix minimizer is called "The Soother". The Soother can be drugs, sex, TV, shopping, gambling. **For an overwhelming number of Americans, it's FOOD**.

Here's the difficult thing about The Soother...It works! It does indeed diminish the pain. Temporarily.

You can see how a habit or an addiction can easily be formed without you ever being aware you are moving down a very slippery path.

After The Soother has taken hold, you have two problems instead of one. The original hurt is still an unhealed wound, and you have a habit which inhibits you from progress.

You may have accumulated <u>many</u> unhealed hurts. You could be using the same Soother or a variety. Juggling the original pain(s) and the Soother(s) demands an increase of frequency and intensity of addictive behavior.

The good news is that you don't have to examine all the hurts, revisit and try to treat the wounds one by one. You just need to reconnect the once healthy system that is still intact but interrupted. Some dynamic results are available by rebalancing your personal story which you repeat to yourself over and again - the story which keeps you running faster and faster, but staying in place.

Dynamically rebalancing your system will empower you to consciously rewrite your script. When you embrace the process of change, you reconnect with your natural balance and life enthusiasm.

Dynamic Rebalancing involves mental, physiological, social, spiritual, and emotional intervention. A guide takes you through the process.

If you are interested in learning more about Dynamic Rebalancing, contact JJFitness at www.JJFitness.net

If you have a day during the 12 weeks that you eat a 1 or 2 on the Perfect 6 Scale:

Describe your thoughts/feelings Before, During and After you broke your healthy eating plan with unhealthy food/alcohol.

Before

During

After

Especially if you're really struggling to stay on track with your eating plan, take a few days and record in your Discovery Journal <u>everything</u> you eat. The heightened sense of awareness that what you put in your body is responsible for your state of being will be in front of you in black and white.

If you are overweight, working out in a gym can be a difficult environment. Here are a few things to remember:

Health and Fitness are abstract states, only sometimes are their signs visible.

People can appear to be fit who are not.

People can be fit who do not appear to be so.

Here are a few things to remember about working out and eating well.

As your fitness level increases, so does your energy level!

Training does not get easier as one becomes more fit.

Quitting sugar can be as hard as quitting smoking...Hang In There!

And speaking of persistence: You lose weight the same way you put it on - one pound at a time.

To lose weight and keep it off you must be at your best every day. But if for one reason or another you're not, ACT LIKE YOU ARE!!!

Assertive trainees are intense, confident and persistent.

These qualities are a result of **overcoming** the difficult challenges you set.

When you don't meet a challenge, it is often due to a lack of commitment and discipline.

Re-commit and establish enough discipline for the period of the new challenge.

JJ's Way 5 Steps to Get Back in ACTION

1. Make a RE-commitment. For the next 8 weeks, you are going to follow the JJ's Way eating plan!
2. You are going to rid your kitchen of your forbidden foods
3. You are going to limit your Sugar and Starch intake
4. You will drink lots of water
5. You will become fit and learn the basics of resistance training.

Remember this:

An increased metabolism is a <u>pleasurable</u> feeling.

Controlled insulin and reduced insulin resistance makes weight loss EASY.

Chapter 15: Weeks 9 - 12 Training

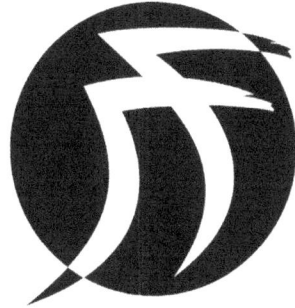

Your explorations of the past TWO MONTHS have energized you, filling you with new confidence and inspiration.

Challenges are becoming more welcome than a familiar routine used to be!

You are developing awareness and intuition.

There is no choice but to keep going!

Again, note that the exercises on Day 3 are NOT done in supersets.

"NEVER GET COMFORTABLE"

Let's Keep Training!

Indicates "Super Set"	
Indicates "Hara" exercise	

DAY ONE

PAGE	ACTIVITY	REPS	SETS	BREAK
67	Warm up	5 min	Zone 1	
81	Toe Touches	8	2	no break
83	DB Lateral Raise	12		
84	DB Military Press	12	3	60 sec
89	Front Hold	30 sec		
87	Hip Raise	40 sec	2	30 sec
94	DB Chest Press	12		
96	Band Flye	12	3	60 sec
106	Push ups	10 to 12		
91	Modified Leg Raise	15	3	no break
79	Cardio	25 min	Intervals	
67	Cool down	5 min	Zone 1	
69	Stretch	5 min		

DAY TWO
Rest and Diet

DAY THREE

PAGE	ACTIVITY	REPS	SETS	BREAK
67	Warm up	5 min	Zone 1	
92	Side Bends	10 sec	3	no break
101	Band Squat	12	3	30 - 10 sec
85	Band Stationary Lunge	12	3	30 - 10 sec
90	Calf Raise	15	3	30 - 10 sec
103	Quad Extension with arm	60 sec	2	10 sec
112	Step Ups	24	3	30 - 10 sec
115	Single Leg Lateral Lift	12	3	30 - 10 sec
125	Romanian DB Pull	12	3	30 - 10 sec
108	Crossovers	15	3	no break
79	Cardio	25 min	Zone 2	
67	Cool down	5 min	Zone 1	
69	Stretch	8 min		

DAY FOUR

PAGE	ACTIVITY	REPS	SETS	BREAK
67	Warm up	5 min	Zone 1	
81	Toe Touches	8	2	no break
114	Pulldown	12		
109	Low Row	12	3	30 - 10 sec
110	Pullover	12		
113	Bridge Track	8	2	30 Sec
105	Band Curls	5 hold 10		
137	DB Hammer Curl	10	3	30 - 10 sec
138	Tricep Extension	12		
118	Frog Leg Crunch	15	3	no break
119	Sprinter stretch	20 sec	2	no break
79	Cardio	25 min	Zone 2	
67	Cool down	5 min	Zone 1	
69	Stretch	5 min		

DAY FIVE
Rest and Diet

DAY SIX

PAGE	ACTIVITY	REPS	SETS	BREAK
67	Warm up	5 min	Zone 1	
121	Tip Toe Track	10	2	20 sec
122	Donkey Kick	12	3	30 sec
139	1 Arm DB Military Press	12	3	30 sec
127	4 point balance	1 min	2	10 sec
140	1 Arm DB Chest Press	12		
141	Jump Rope	30-60 sec	3	30 - 10 sec
123	Dips	12		
130	Plank	60 sec	2	10 sec
131	Tree Pose	2 min	1	
79	Cardio	20 min	Intervals	
67	Cool down	5 min	Zone 1	
69	Stretch	5 min		

DAY SEVEN
Rest and Diet

Now is the moment of truth. Only you know how well you've followed the course.

Like we did on Day 1, measure the following body parts with a tape measure and write them in your Discovery Journal:

Shoulders:

Chest:

Waist:

Hips:

Mid Thigh (right):

Upper Arm (right):

Wrist (right):

In the morning, before you've eaten, step on the scale (make sure it is the same scale!) and write down your weight in your Discovery Journal. Take two Front and Side pictures, print them, and tape them in your Journal.

Look back to the first pages in your Journal. What are the differences? How do you feel?

Chapter 16: What's Next?

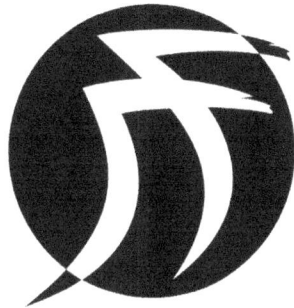

If you have made it through 3 MONTHS, you have discovered everything you need for the continuing journey.

You have made it!

| *"WINNING IS A HABIT"* | The determination you have developed can help you meet ALL your goals. |

Determination is a tool of winners.

Contact JJFitness for Information about the <u>Discovery of JJ's Way DVD</u> and the next JJ's Way books, <u>Reaching Your Goal Weight JJ's Way</u> and <u>The Complete JJ's Way Guide to Nutrition</u>.

Come to JJFitness.net and feel the spirit of health, wellness and unity.

www.JJFitness.net

I wish you the best of luck on your Fitness Journey.

Fitness is a state of being: Just Be Fit!

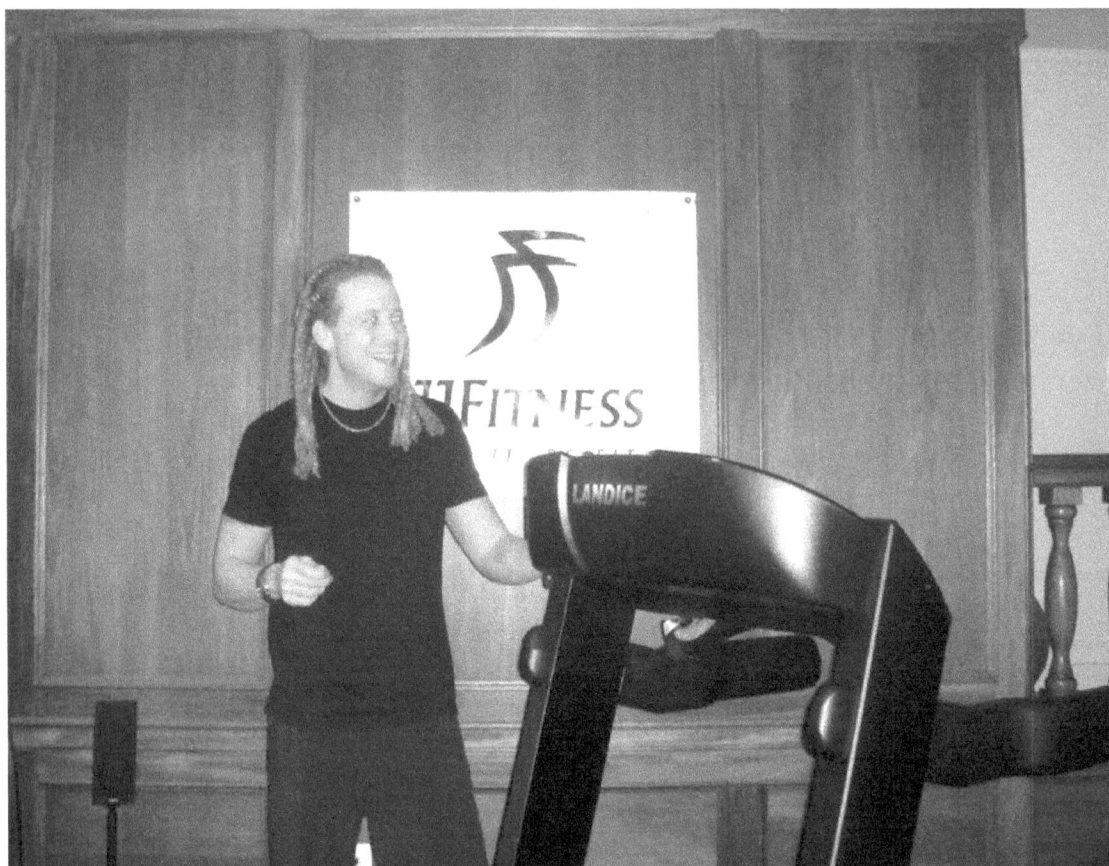

About JJ

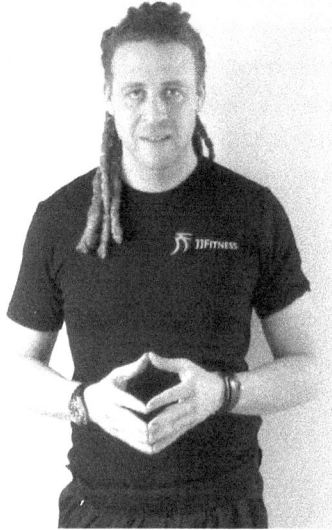

JJ is the founder of JJFitness and one of the premier strength and conditioning trainers in the country.

Based in Howard County, Maryland at a private, state-of-the-art fitness facility, JJ's diverse clientele range from professional and amateur athletes to dedicated individuals from all walks of life, from onscreen entertainers to corporate executives, all of whom have achieved greater personal and professional success from **JJ's Way**, an integrated mind and body training approach.

JJ is a master of exercise form and intensity; his innovative training philosophies have made him *the* most sought after fitness expert for those who expect immediate and real results.

Certified as a Performance Enhancement Specialist by the National Association of Sports Medicine (NASM) and by the American Council of Exercise (ACE), JJ brings more than 15 years of skills and experience as a former athlete, scholar, and teacher into his current fitness consulting practice.

JJ holds multiple degrees from Cornell University and University of California, Berkeley. His true dedication, skillful motivation, and real application of the mind/body connection make him a truly unique standout in the preparation for THE NEXT LEVEL of fitness and wellness.

www.ingramcontent.com/pod-product-compliance
Lightning Source LLC
Chambersburg PA
CBHW081153270326

41930CB00014B/3137